"*Lisa was in life about as brave a soul as y*
now she's left her words of courage to help ot
Inspiring, brave and giving describe Lisa, i
that up."

JOHN CALDWELL, CEO - RWR GROUP

"*The day I met Lisa – Melbourne Cup Day 2016 – is etched on my mind.
Lisa had that X factor; she oozed confidence even when she was stricken with
unimaginable pain.*

*Reading the book, I felt like I got to know Lisa even more: her resilience,
her battle and her never-give-up attitude is a running theme throughout what
is one of the most emotional, bittersweet, sad but weirdly uplifting books about
a young woman who, with the help and love of her family and friends, lived
like a rockstar until she took her last breath.*

*Lisa, quite seriously, will never be forgotten. I could not put the book down
and read it in one session – yes, she left that kind of mark. Wherever her spirit
is now, she will be singing, dancing, joking and still working out what she
should wear to her next Melbourne Cup VIP appearance.*

*Lisa rocked. She made the most of the cards she had been dealt and boy,
was a mighty fine rockstar until she left this world. I could not put the book
down – it really is a must-read. Love you, Lisa. And Mumma, Geraldine, you
are just as big a shining light as your exquisite daughter.*"

MELISSA HOYER
Media Editor and Commentator, News Corporation & Seven Network
Sunrise, The Morning Show and The Daily Edition

"*Like any iconic tale, I knew what was coming and how it would end, yet I
couldn't put it down and loved every minute of it. I can't remember a book
that has given me so many constant streams of tears whilst also giving me
literal laugh-out-very-loud moments. It's beautifully co-written both from the
point of view of a dying daughter and a mother watching her loved one die.*

*It's a must-read for anyone feeling like their life needs perspective, craving
a tale that will move them at their very core. It's an emotional manual for
anyone on a cancer journey, whether they are the one coping with cancer or a
loved one supporting.*"

CONSTANCE HALL, BLOGGER AND AUTHOR

Kudos by the Terminally Fabulous Rockstars

www.terminallyfabulous.com

"It's a testament to how much you have affected so many, Lisa, with your honesty and at times harrowing account of this hideous disease. I pray you are comfortable and know that so many here have you in their thoughts. Be proud of yourself for sharing this journey with us, and I hope we have at times helped you along the way. You are an inspiration to so many, Lisa. If we can be half as amazing as you in life, then we are blessed."

SHARON PECK

"You are my inspiration even though we have different cancers. Hearing and reading your blog helps us to keep fighting even when we have been given the worst news ever from our oncologists. Your humour and wit are fab. You make us all smile, cry and laugh out loud and wish that we could be there for you. It's amazing how many hearts YOU have touched, ROCKSTAR."

MAYANA WILSON

"Keep fighting, our inspiring, strong and truly amazing fighter ... You are still here for a reason. You continue to inspire. You continue to change lives. Your mission isn't finished yet. I desperately want you out of pain. Your friends that have gone before went with you in their hearts. Don't forget that."

SIMONE LEIGH

"Here you are still finding the energy to let us all know what's happening. I don't think I know of any of the correct words to describe how amazing you are to all of us and how inspirational you have been to me personally. THANK YOU."

JULES JULES

"Lisa, you are a beautiful person, with an even more beautiful soul. You can make me laugh then cry in an instant. I'm angry for you. I'm sad for your loved ones, and yet I'm happy that I have found your blog as you have made me a better person..."

LISA SUTHERLAND TAYLOR

"You are truly inspiring. As a person dying from end stage lung disease, you have me thinking differently. The timelines are what we make. Every day is a gift to be made the most of."

MARNIE PENGELLY

"You are one amazing woman and are teaching me so much about really living and being real. Just love you."

SHEILA WEDEGIS

"Your transparency is awe inspiring and breathtaking, sadly not in the fabulous pair of shoes kind of way but an altogether different way. I want to thank you for your magnificent courage and eternal gift of words. You inspire me every day to laugh louder, love harder and live longer."

SIOUX WHITTAKER

"What an amazing woman you are! You are the chief Rockstar after all. Sending love to you all."

CHRISTINE SMITH

"I am so relieved to be reading this blog while sitting propped up in my bed. I am only just starting my terminal journey, but your writing, humour and, best of all, honesty make me realise I will be able to give as best a fight as I can to this b****rd and will not be afraid. I respect you and admire you so much for still giving to others while everything else seems to be being taken away from you and your family."

JOANNE JAGGER

"Is it wrong for me to say a goodbye now? The fear when I see a post from you in case it's written on your behalf and I've missed my chance to say it as I thought it may be in bad taste. You are both amazing and heartbreakingly honest. To say I will miss your posts and humour is an understatement. Love to you Lisa and to all who know you."

REBECCA INGRAM

"Dear God, Lisa, we're all faced with a terrible dilemma. We want your pain to end but fear what that will bring. And words fail me. They just seem so inadequate to summarise the love and support we're all so desperate to show you all. Wishing you a bit of respite and quality time with loved ones."

THOMAS WILTON-RUMNEY

"I know it's different, Lisa, but my mum is my only friend and she is 84, and I make sure I see her every day. Most importantly, I ring her every night before she goes to bed so in my heart, I know that if there is no tomorrow that I had that last conversation with her and that she knows I love her. We all love you, Lisa, and I hope you can feel that love. My words won't make a difference but thank you for being the amazing woman you are."

SHARRON REDMOND

"You know you've done this in spades, yeah? You should be incredibly proud of what you've done, and what you continue to do, even when you're feeling like shit! You're the Rockstariest Rockstar, Lisa!"

HELEN LACY

TERMINALLY
fabulous

A young woman's fight for dignity and fabulousness
on her terminal cancer journey

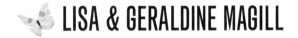 LISA & GERALDINE MAGILL

Terminally Fabulous: A young woman's fight for dignity and fabulousness on her terminal cancer journey

Author – Lisa and Geraldine Magill
www.terminallyfabulous.com
Terminally.Fabulous35@gmail.com
© Geraldine Magill 2019

If the reader requires assistance on the cancer journey, please refer to a list of resources and organisations at the end of this book.

Cover Image:
"Fearless"
From the Lisa Magill Collection
by Hayley Walker
www.hayleywalkerart.com

Instagram: Hayleyswalkerart
Instagram: Manifestationartist
Facebook: Hayley Walker Art

Editing and Publishing Support: www.AuthorSupportServices.com

ISBN: 978-0-6483917-1-5 (pbk) 978-0-6483917-8-4 (hbk)

A catalogue record for this book is available from the National Library of Australia

This book is dedicated to every cancer sufferer, past and present, and anyone affected by this nightmare disease. There is no such thing as losing the fight. The true strength of a warrior is battling until the end, be it cure or passing. Love and utmost respect always.

About the Author

Lisa Magill

> *"Lisa loved the idea of leaving something behind. She wanted*
> *to help anyone she met. This book ensures that happens now,*
> *long after she has gone."*
>
> – Geraldine Magill

Lisa navigated the minefield that is cancer just after turning 30 years old. Her friends, family and colleagues had told her for years that she should put her thoughts into words. Four years into her journey with cancer, she decided to begin. Heartbreakingly honest, raw and direct in her writing, Lisa tells you her story with no holds barred.

She didn't write her blog to offer enlightenment. There was no motive to make you radically change your diet and start chanting at a full moon.

She wrote the blog for her.

And for her family.

Geraldine Magill

> *"I really do love you, Geraldine, and I'm so thankful for you,*
> *because no-one else would put up with me."*
>
> – Lisa Magill

Geraldine is a mother, wife, friend and also a daughter herself. She travelled this difficult road right alongside her daughter, Lisa, throughout the good, the bad and the ugly side of all things cancer.

For those people coping with cancer and wondering if you are still normal... yes, you are still normal. Lisa and Geraldine have shared their private thoughts and moments to redefine that word for you.

Acknowledgements

Heartfelt thanks to our family and friends near and far, whose love and support never faltered day or night during the most difficult of times.

Special thanks to Di Olson, a stranger who reached out at the beginning of this book writing journey. She listened, she advised, and she was always there when I most needed her. Di introduced me to the amazing Alex Fullerton and her talented team of editors without whom this book would not have come to fruition. I not only met an amazing group of experts, but I have gained lifelong friends.

To every Terminally Fabulous Rockstar, you were there for Lisa as you have been for me and my family throughout our heartbreaking journey. You comforted Lisa through the longest nights when she was wracked with pain and gave her the strength that she needed to make it through each life-threatening event. She loved you all dearly for it; we all did. We are eternally grateful.

To every medical professional we came in contact with, we were so blessed to meet each of you at the right time and stage of Lisa's cancer journey. Lisa would never forgive me if I didn't make a special mention of the following people, who were our knights in shining armour when we most needed you:

Dr Fenton-Lee, Lisa's surgeon – Your caring and supportive approach during the longest of waits was faultless.

Dr Martin Tattersall, Lisa's much-loved and favourite oncologist – You were the one that gave her hope when there was none

Dr Warren Joubert and Dr David Pryor, the oncologist and radiologist who were with us during the final stages of Lisa's cancer journey – You never gave up looking for new treatments and revisiting old treatments to complement Lisa's fighting spirit. You gave us more time to make unforgettable memories. Without you both Lisa would not have made it to her 35th year.

The Palliative Care Team at Ipswich General Hospital – The level of care, love and support you gave to Lisa and our family were second to none. You gave Lisa the peace of mind and comfort she needed to allow her to pass without the fear she had carried around for so long. Your words of advice and support helped our family get through the darkest of days.

Dr Ross Cruikshank – The heartfelt respect and dignity you gave Lisa until the very end touched our hearts and gave us peace of mind when we most needed it.

Each and every one of you are angels in disguise. We will never be able to thank you for all you have done. We remain forever indebted to you.

Dr Jodie Ross, Lisa's amazing GP – Not only did you provide Lisa with the best advice and care possible, you also recognised our family struggles and heartbreak and ensured we were aware of the support mechanisms available to help us deal with them. Your availability day or night and your many home visits were welcomed by us all, just knowing we were being heard and receiving your words of wisdom gave us the peace of mind needed to get through another day, we all loved you for it.

Last but by no means least, to our beautiful granddaughter Ava. You will never know the difference you made to each of us when we most needed it. The love, care and adoration you showered on your Aunty Lisa was endearing to the end. You were definitely a gift from God. We count our blessings every day.

Geraldine Magill
Lisa's mother

www.terminallyfabulous.com

Contents

Introduction

"Always remember, you are braver
than you think, stronger than you seem
and loved more than you know."

-Christopher Robin (A.A. Milne)

The 11th of March 2017 is a date we will never forget. This date will be remembered by our family, friends and thousands of people around the world. It was the day we all knew was coming – the day our beautiful daughter Lisa died.

Most of these people had never met Lisa, yet they knew every intimate detail of the final 13 months of her cancer journey, in her own words, 'the good the bad and the ugly'. Lisa had started a blog, *Terminally Fabulous,* to record her journey with terminal cancer. She blogged brutally and honestly about her experiences, and ours, and quickly had an audience of thousands of people worldwide. She was open and forthright and never backed down from giving her opinion on things. This gave permission for others in her situation to feel however they felt. She normalised the cancer experience for people who had nothing to hold onto.

When Lisa decided to start a blog, I had mixed feelings. I definitely thought it would be good for her psychologically, and secretly I believed it would give me a better insight into how she was truly feeling. However, I was also worried. I worried about how Lisa, and our family, would be perceived and, being completely transparent, I was worried about the content. Lisa was never one for holding back. If you upset or annoyed her you knew about it, and not in the most discreet manner. Lisa believed honesty was the best policy, and at times her honesty could be scathing.

I already knew what Lisa felt about me on any given day (on any given hour and minute, actually), but the thought of everyone else knowing was frightening. Locked in a world of pain, medication and frustration, the only thing Lisa felt she had any control over were her words. At the time, I constantly wore a coat of armour for protection. I knew when she was venting her frustrations in the moment and that her opinion would change within an hour or two, but the public would not know this. At times, depending on what the blog subject was, I was sure it would cause extra stress on an already stressful situation.

Lisa offered to stop the blog when she saw how upsetting her words could be at times. But knowing we might be helping another person or family to realise that what they were going through was normal made me determined to feel the fear and do it anyway. The ongoing messages from readers saying they'd been helped immensely by our honesty and experience convinced me that what Lisa was doing was positive.

It's that thought that led to this 'warts-and-all' book. I sincerely hope that by reading this collection of Lisa's blog posts, and my thoughts, people will continue to be helped. I hope that you, if you're living with or caring for someone with terminal cancer, receive comfort from knowing what our journey was like. As Lisa had said, "I want this blog to give different perspectives because, at the end of the day, it's not all about me. Cancer affects everyone around you".

It's by talking about the good, the bad and the ugly that we keep ourselves sane and keep the unimaginably heartrending experience manageable. During our nightmare journey, I could somehow suppress all my feelings and emotions. I had to; it was my coping mechanism. It was like I was an outsider playing a part in someone else's life. I was doing the right things and saying the right things. Looking back, though, I can't even recognise myself. How could I even consider stopping the blog when thousands of families were going through the same thing and looking for answers and support – anything to get them through the day?

Many of the blog followers, the Terminally Fabulous Rockstars, asked Lisa to write a book. They loved her humour, wit and passion for life. When she laughed they laughed, and when she cried they cried. And they wanted more. Lisa and I talked about it many times. She loved the idea of leaving something behind, and she wanted to give back to those who had given to her so selflessly. She also wanted to help anyone she met, and the book would ensure this happened long after she was gone. Sadly, time was against us. Lisa had the vision, but her energy was fading by the day and talk of a book was eventually shelved. All her energy was needed to get through another day and another blog. I am so pleased that now I can fulfil Lisa's desire to publish this book based on her very honest and real *Terminally Fabulous* blogs. And this is also a way to ensure Lisa's voice continues to be heard.

Following each blog, I share my reflection as her mother and 24/7 carer. It's my way to fill in the blanks and to raise awareness for other carers. I have also provided a list of organisations and resources recommended by Lisa and myself at the back of this book to be of further assistance for families on the cancer journey. Please, reach out when you need help. You don't have to be alone on this path.

For those that knew Lisa and read her blog, this book will remind you of our happiest and saddest times. You'll also learn a little more of what our family went though.

I hope that through this book you will also realise how much she thought of you and your support as the end drew near. When she told you all in her final video that you gave her strength and determination to keep fighting, it wasn't just words. You always found the right words to help her through another tough day, whether it was to thank her for helping you through your own journey or just to pass on your love and admiration. She was in awe of you all.

For those new to *Terminally Fabulous*, I hope this book gives you a true insight into what it's like to live your final months knowing how your story will end. My daughter Lisa fought long and hard every day. I now know why others refer to those that are fighting cancer as heroes. Lisa's pain was unbearable, the treatments horrendous and her fear of dying heart-wrenching. But her spirit and determination to see another day were relentless.

For those going through their own terminal journey, I hope that by sharing our experience you feel you are not alone, whether you are the patient, parent, sibling, family member or friend. I truly hope we give you some of the answers you've been looking for, or the comfort you need during your most challenging days.

"It's simple; I'm in love with life and to die is to take away my greatest love."

–Lisa Magill

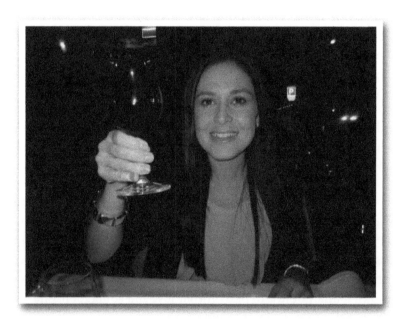

13 August 2011
Lisa Magill.

2001

Walking through the departure gates at Sydney airport to return to Ireland for a few years was one of the hardest things we had ever done. We were leaving our girl behind, at her own choice. Lisa, 19 years old, was crying on one side of the glass doors and we the same on the other. We nearly turned back but somehow kept going.

This is something I think we will regret for as long as we live. What we would give to have those extra five years with Lisa.

If only we'd known what lay ahead.

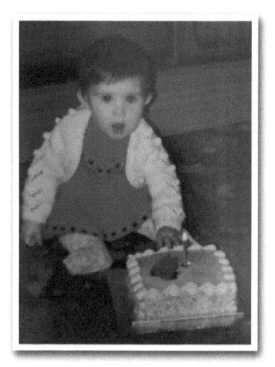

Lisa, aged one.

Lisa, aged ten, and
Steven, aged eight.

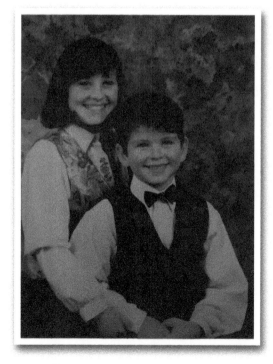

Life BC: Before Cancer

Lisa doesn't mention much about our family life pre-diagnosis in her *Terminally Fabulous* blogs. But a life is so much more than just a diagnosis, as you'll see...

We had first emigrated to Australia from Ireland when Lisa was eight and Steven was five. Although we had no family here, we had a couple of friends who helped us get settled. From the minute we landed in this country we all loved it. It was the lifestyle we had always wanted for our family. Lisa missed family back home but always proudly described herself as an Aussie.

Lisa was a strong-willed, independent child with great determination, whose temperament didn't change much at all as she grew. Once she made up her mind, no-one could change it.

She was the child who'd come home from school and do her homework without being asked. Her brother Steven was the opposite; he wrote the little black book of homework excuses and was proud of it. Like most siblings Lisa and Steven fought, but pity the person who looked sideways at Steven when Lisa was around. She'd have their guts for garters. Though she was small, she was mighty.

We settled into our Australian life in Sydney with a huge amount of support from friends who became our family. Like most families, we went from year to year working, parenting our growing children, celebrating landmarks like birthdays and Christmas and taking the children to the theme parks they loved. Lisa always enjoyed the hair-raising rides, which she went on with her dad. Steven and I kept to the smaller rides and screamed like our lives depended on it.

I don't know a family who hasn't had teen troubles at some point. We were no different. We moved through the boyfriend phase, which was heartbreaking to watch. Then came the smoking phase where Lisa, who'd had asthma continually as a child, decided to take up smoking and was sprung by me late one night. What a fright I gave her when I turned on a downstairs light and surprised her, puffing away through the open French doors!

Lisa managed to achieve the marks to get into criminal psychology at university, but she decided to take a gap year. She never did go back to study, no matter how much we encouraged her. Instead, she found a position at an optometrist's and settled into working there. She'd had her confidence knocked by a harrowing break-up with a boyfriend, and despite our cajoling, we had to accept that she would do things in her own time.

When Lisa was 19, Peter and I decided to move back to Ireland for four or five years to be with our parents while they were still with us and in somewhat good health. Our plan was to sell up and take Lisa and Steven with us. As much as we knew Lisa could take care of herself, we thought the fresh start would be good for her. Spending time with her cousins and doing a bit of travel while we were so close to Europe ... Who could say no to that? Lisa, that's who. She refused to uproot her life for those years. So, we decided to find her a place to live, help set her up and hopefully find someone reliable to share with her, which we did.

The closer the day of the big move came, the higher our anxiety grew. Even though Lisa was clear on her intention to stay in Australia, Peter and I secretly hoped she would change her mind at the last minute. But we were kidding ourselves. Once Lisa set her mind on something, there was no changing it.

Walking through the departure gates at Sydney airport was one of the hardest things we had ever done. Lisa was crying on one side of the glass doors and we on the other. We were so close to turning back but somehow kept going. This is something I think we will regret for as long as we live. What we would give to have those extra five years with Lisa. If only we'd known what lay ahead.

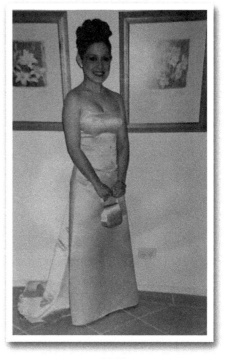

2001
Lisa at home in Claremont Meadows, NSW, before her Year 12 Formal.

While we were away, Lisa found a new boyfriend who was so much older than her that, at first, she wouldn't tell us his age. Knowing her determination, all we could do was watch and hope that all would be well as she gave up her job to work with him in a government department. As time passed, it was apparent that he wasn't everything we hoped for our daughter.

From her guarded words, I got a very uneasy feeling about the relationship. Occasionally, she would say things that led me to believe he was controlling and rather a tyrant. From across the globe, I worried for her and couldn't think of anything positive that could come from this. Perhaps it's natural as her mother, but all I could think about were the things that she would miss out on: the big white wedding, building a first home together and children. He'd been married before and already had a family.

From that distance, and with the powerlessness of a parent of adult children, I had to accept that as much as you love your kids and want to support

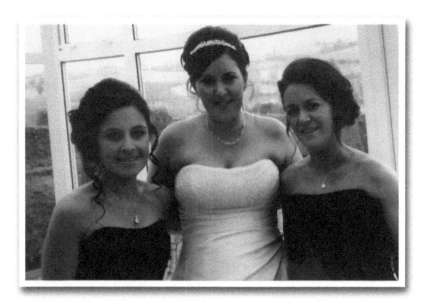

11 December 2010
Lisa, new sister-in-law Marianne and Paula Folliard in Co. Derry, Northern
Ireland, on Steven (Lisa's brother) and Marianne's wedding day

them, it's impossible to accept all their choices. Still, as hard as you try to let them grow up, you can't help but want to protect them. We persevered, spoke often and insisted on paying for her to come over and visit us, so we could spend some time with her every now and again. I think we were all relieved, though, when we decided to move back Down Under.

Peter and I chose Brisbane to settle in this time. Sydney is beautiful but extremely fast paced, and it is so spread out and congested that driving from A to B is a nightmare. Thankfully, we loved our new life in Brisbane. We were both working, bought a lovely home and got ourselves settled.

Steven had met Marianne back in Ireland, and they decided to move to Australia to spend a year with us. Unbeknown to us this was a tester for Marianne to see if she could move away to the other side of the world, leaving her friends and family and everything familiar back home. The test was a success and we rejoiced! Having the family back in one country meant the world to us.

She would dance like no-one was watching.

We saw Lisa often. She would fly up with her partner for weekends here and there, and on the rare occasion, she would come on her own. These were our favourite visits as we would see glimpses of the 18-year-old Lisa we all knew and loved shining through, always smiling, relaxed and happy to socialise. After a couple of glasses of champagne, she would dance like no-one was watching and was always the life and soul of the party. Her one-liners would come one after the other, and we often hoped she would cancel her flight home and stay with us in Brisbane.

Lisa had been diagnosed as coeliac by this time too. She'd had digestive troubles for a while and going gluten-free seemed to help. I thought it quite unusual for a young woman of her age to need medication to move her bowels, but we just accepted it as something Lisa needed. It was only

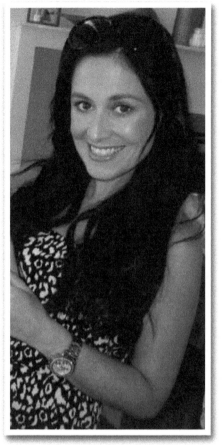

2010
Lisa, pre-cancer, visiting friends in Forster.

later that we wondered whether this diagnosis was linked in any way with the one that was to come.

Lisa's relationship continued to be fraught. Her visits to us were often made difficult as she was bombarded with telephone calls from her partner who, Lisa told us, did not like her socialising without him. More and more, we saw Lisa ending her evenings in tears, shutting herself into her room for whispered phone conversations as she was barraged with questions as to who she was with, what she was doing and where she had been. This controlling behaviour was alarming.

Over time, Lisa lost friends over the relationship. Her inability to have girly catch-ups without boyfriend drama hampered many a friendship. Thankfully, she had some close friends who stood by her, even though they didn't see her as often as they'd like. As long as there was enough contact for them to know she was safe, that was all that mattered to them. They were aware of my worries for Lisa and would often put my mind at ease if I called, concerned about a recent argument.

It was only in the last 18 months of Lisa's life that we discovered just how controlling he truly was. It was terrifying. Lisa shared how he would hide her phone, handbag and car keys to keep her from having contact with everyone that knew her. She said he would play mind games, convincing her that he was the only one that cared for her. For some reason he gave her the hardest time about her relationship with her dad. He would try and turn things Peter had said in love into some perverted comment and make out that Peter had ulterior motives.

Although Lisa believed some of what he said at times, she never let him impact her relationship with us, her family. The harder he tried, the more she resisted. She began to realise just how far he would go to keep her isolated from everyone that cared for her. Her fear and his manipulation kept her with him for too long. It was to be one of her greatest regrets.

March 2012

Lisa came up to Queensland to spend a couple of weeks with us. It was rare enough that she got to come alone, but this time it was for two weeks! We were so excited to see her. During this trip, Lisa encouraged me to go for a daily walk, having listened to me moan and complain about my weight for years. Lisa enjoyed exercise. Being just 4 foot 11 inches, and loving rich foods and fine champagne, she did all she could to maintain her tiny frame. I, on the other hand, preferred to whine whilst hoping the fat would magically disappear.

After one of our walks, Lisa mentioned a lump on her side that she had noticed had grown dramatically over the past few months and was starting to become uncomfortable. She pulled up her top to show me. I couldn't believe she hadn't mentioned it before. It was just below her ribs on the left-hand side and was easily 12 centimetres long by 5 centimetres wide. I tried to reassure her that it was probably nothing but strongly suggested she needed to go straight to her doctor when back in Sydney. She had an amazing GP who would get to the bottom of it in no time.

During this trip, Lisa talked about leaving her partner and moving up to Queensland. We were all secretly hoping she would see it through, but we weren't overly-optimistic as we'd heard her say these things before. All we could do was live in hope.

For the rest of the visit, I couldn't get the thought of the lump out of my head. I felt more uneasy than usual when it was time for Lisa to leave. She promised me that she would make an appointment with her GP as soon as she got back to Sydney.

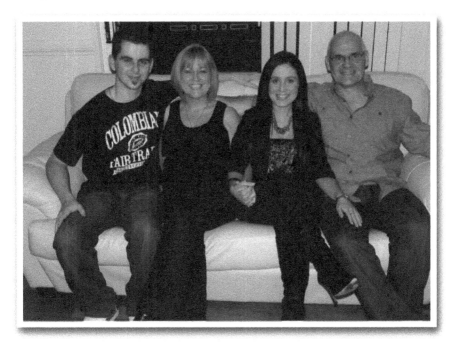

August 2010
Steven, Geraldine, Lisa and Peter Magill at their home in Springfield
Lakes, QLD, during Lisa's visit home for Mum and Dad's birthdays.

The C-Word: Round One

I remember the day of Lisa's appointment clearly. I was watching the clock, trying to imagine what was going on. It was like time was standing still; each minute seemed to take an hour. When Lisa called, she was on her way to get a scan. Her doctor suspected the lump was a tumour. Although Lisa sounded a little frightened, I don't think the enormity of the situation had sunk in.

Once again, I went straight into Mum-Mode and encouraged her not to think too far ahead until she got the results. Something inside me, however, knew our lives were about to change forever.

Things moved fast. The scans confirmed her doctor's suspicions, and within days Lisa was booked in to have the tumour removed. They found it was extremely large and exceedingly rare. It baffled the pathology departments in Australia, so they sent a sample to the US for further testing.

Lisa was in hospital for four weeks because the medical team hadn't been able to get her stomach to work again after the surgery. Thankfully, with the help of medication, she was able to eat small amounts frequently, enough to give her body the goodness it needed to heal her wounds and go home. But by the time she got home, her weight had dropped to 37 kilograms. She was never big before, but now she looked so thin and weak.

We didn't realise that this was only the beginning.

If you've ever waited on pathology results, you'd know that it is an emotional rollercoaster. One day we would be positive, telling Lisa we had a good feeling that things were going to be okay. And the next we'd hide away from her, fearful she would see how upset and worried we were. Lisa was no different. She would switch from being in the best mood to the depths of despair in a matter of minutes. It was unbearable to watch. We would ring the doctor frequently, asking if the pathology results were back.

It seemed to take forever. Six weeks after the surgery, on one of our regular calls, he told us that if the tumour had been benign the results would be back by now. That was his way of telling us to be prepared, I suspect. That's one thing we never did learn to do. With every test, every scan and every new treatment, we would live in hope for good news. Preparing for disappointment was out of the question.

Finally, nine weeks after surgery the results were back. Lisa was diagnosed with undifferentiated gastrointestinal sarcoma. In other words, a type of tumour that had never been seen before, which they didn't know how to treat. We were devastated. Lisa cried on and off for over a week; we all did.

Why was this happening to us? Why Lisa and not Peter or me? We'd rather it was us than her. There was no rhyme or reason.

Lisa was referred to an oncologist. Although the tumour had been removed, it was discovered during testing that there was evidence of disease on the margins of the tumour. Further surgery would be required, along with chemo to give Lisa the best chance possible of beating this cruel disease.

We had loved dealing with Lisa's original surgeon. He showed a genuine concern for Lisa's welfare and continued to stay in contact throughout her cancer journey. Unfortunately, we can't say the same for her first oncologist. He was not far off retirement and talked about it constantly rather than about Lisa's condition and treatment options. At times I felt as though Lisa was the doctor as she did more exploration for potential treatments and surgeries than her oncologist. She asked so many questions and read up as much as possible on her cancer and current treatments. She was always the first to clarify the barrage of medical terms thrown at us and somehow was an expert at simplifying it for the rest of us to understand. We couldn't have been prouder of her.

It was agreed that Lisa would have a combination of doxorubicin and gemcitabine, both powerful chemotherapy drugs. She was also to have Neulasta, a self-administered drug to boost white cell count and reduce infection risk, which she'd have to inject into her stomach. As scary as it was, Lisa was prepared to go to any lengths to give herself the best possible chance of survival.

She was warned that due to the toxicity of the chemotherapies, her nurses would be dressed in protective suits and plastic face masks. I don't think anything could have prepared us for this. They were like something from a sci-fi movie. To think that this chemical stuff would be pumped into our beautiful girl's veins was terrifying. Thankfully, the nurses were wonderful. They did their very best to put Lisa's mind at ease and to ensure she was fully aware of the after-effects of the treatment and how to deal with them.

I'd often heard that the treatment of cancer can be as bad as its symptoms, if not worse. Sadly, it took me to see it with my own eyes to believe it. Lisa was in bed for at least a week after each cycle. The pain and nausea were so bad she would roll into a ball in the middle of the bed, crying out and begging for relief. Her partner would have to carry her to the bathroom, otherwise she would never have made it. As difficult as it is to admit, he did step up to the mark when it came to caring for Lisa after treatment. I don't think anyone else could have done it as well as he did, and it wasn't easy.

Peter and I would travel down for a few days every couple of weeks, but we worried constantly about overstaying our welcome. We wanted to be there every minute of every day for Lisa, but we didn't want to make life any harder for her than it already was. At least we knew her partner was taking good care of her, which was our main concern.

Lisa was torn apart by how changed she looked. She was someone who wouldn't have left the house without the perfect make-up, hair, outfit and matching handbag. Now she was a cancer sufferer with no hair, no eyebrows and that constant grey look – and it was tearing her apart. She longed to be the person she had been. She cringed when she thought back to the times when she'd moan and complain about her figure or her looks. Only now could she finally accept she was beautiful. All she wanted was her health back and to be her old self. It broke our hearts that we couldn't help her.

Never in my life did I ever imagine that I would be injecting my daughter with any type of medication, never mind a cancer drug. I was the parent that would run and hide in the corner whilst Peter calmly took control when the kids had a fall. Yet now when I visited, I was injecting Neulasta into Lisa's stomach without batting an eyelid. Truth be told I would have performed open heart surgery if I thought it would help Lisa get her health back. I just wanted this nightmare to end for her – for us all.

Out of all difficult situations there is good to be had. My relationship with Lisa thankfully grew stronger by the day. We were mother and daughter, but we were now also the best of friends. We could talk about anything: our hopes, our dreams and our fears. We would often laugh at some of the arguments we'd had during her teenage years. I reminded her of the time she decided to leave home when she turned 18. She had packed a bag and asked us to leave her at the train station. I cried sore for the next couple of hours, but then my phone rang. It was Lisa asking me to collect her at the station as none of her friends were around to pick her up. Needless to say it didn't take her long to unpack her things and settle back into her room again. I never thought we would ever laugh about that, but time changes everything.

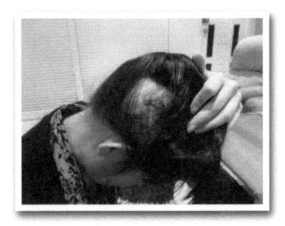

27 July 2012
Lisa starting to lose her hair after chemotherapy. This was heartbreaking for Lisa as she loved her hair.

November 2012

Lisa's chemo was finally completed with the news that there was No Evidence of Disease (NED)! We felt like all our Christmases has come at once. Surely life would go back to normal and our cancer nightmare was behind us. We could start enjoying living again.

How wrong could we be?

The treatment may have ended and the physical impact it had on Lisa's body might have faded in time, but the psychological scars would never be far away. I remember her doctor advising us during Lisa's final consultation to be aware that we would probably all suffer a little PTSD now that the worst was over. I remember looking at him and thinking, *Don't talk silly. Lisa is cured, and we are going to go and put this all behind us. We have a lot of living to do!*

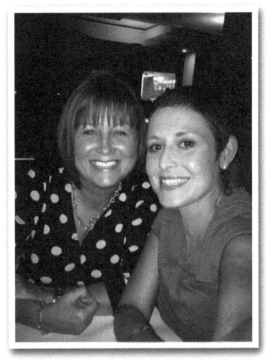

July 2012
Lisa with Geraldine at Doyles Restaurant, Sydney, after shaving her hair.

He was obviously a lot wiser than I gave him credit for. Every little spot, ache or pain sent Lisa into panic mode. What if it was back? What if they missed something in the last scan? As hard as we tried to eliminate her fears it was nearly impossible. How could we ease Lisa of her worries when we were living with the same fears and worries?

Still, as Christmas approached there was a level of excitement I hadn't felt since the kids were young and counting down the days until Santa came.

We were determined to make it special. We had a lot to be thankful for and we were going to celebrate!

A couple of weeks before Christmas, Peter and I had some friends over for an early celebration. We were feeling like life couldn't get any better when the door opened and in walked Steven and Marianne smiling like Cheshire cats. They asked if they could have a quick chat and took us into a bedroom away from our friends. There they told us they were having a baby! How I contained myself that evening without saying anything to our friends I will never know. Our lives couldn't have been any more perfect. We couldn't wait for Lisa to arrive on Christmas Eve to hear the good news.

On the morning she arrived, Lisa seemed in good spirits. She was happy to be joining us for Christmas, but I could tell she wasn't herself. After what she had been through, I wondered if that was even possible. It wasn't long before Steven and Marianne arrived with a small gift for Lisa. They said it wasn't her Christmas gift as they knew Lisa would want to hold off opening it until Christmas morning. She opened it slowly with a confused look on her face. I wanted to grab it from her and rip it open; I so needed to see Lisa happy. Once she realised it was a diamante t-shirt with 'Aunty' written on it she smiled. But we could all tell it was just a surface smile. It wasn't the heartfelt smile you give when something really touches you deep inside.

You could feel the disappointment sit heavy in the room. I'm not sure who was crushed more about her reaction: Steven and Marianne or me. Rather than leave things as is, Steven told her he thought she'd be excited by the news, but she brushed him off. I think this was the moment I realised Lisa would never be her old self.

The next morning Lisa came in and lay beside me in bed. She was deep in thought, and I knew I had to get to the bottom of what was going on. She mentioned Steven questioning her reaction to the pregnancy as if she was confused about what he was expecting. I told her honestly that we were all a little confused at her not being as happy as we'd hoped she'd be. We thought a new baby in the family would be the beautiful distraction we all needed. We hoped it would help us all heal, especially Lisa. She loved kids and was so good with them. That's when she opened up.

Through her tears she explained how she'd heard it said before that when a baby comes into the world, they are sent to replace someone leaving. She believed that someone was her.

You see, that's what cancer does. It not only makes you suffer when you have the disease, the cruelty continues long after the beast has left your body. It sits in the back of your mind and when there is a glimpse of happiness and hope for a brighter future, it pounces with an intensity that you can't explain. It runs deeper than any physical scars it has left behind.

I can't say it was the Christmas I was hoping for. The elephant in the room was constantly lurking, with each of us trying to deal with what we'd been through, especially Lisa. She wanted to believe the worst was over for her, but she was traumatised. Nothing we could do or say was going to help ease her fears.

How could it when we were feeling just as traumatised as her? We tried to encourage her to seek counselling, but she wouldn't hear of it. She had tried it many years ago but didn't have a great experience and had vowed she would never go back.

Time and experience are great teachers. Looking back now, I feel that if Lisa had given counselling a second go early on in her cancer journey, she may have found someone she connected with who could help her. Connecting well with a counsellor can change everything, as I have learned through my own experiences.

Connecting well with a counsellor can change everything.

As Marianne's pregnancy progressed, Lisa began to feel slightly better in herself. Although her demons never left her, she learnt how to deal with them a little more. She even allowed herself to look to the future. She'd talk about travelling to the many places she wanted to go and see. This was her second chance at life and she was determined to make the most of it.

To keep her mind busy, I asked if she would help me with organising the baby shower. After some initial hesitancy, she did what Lisa does best and took full control. I went from being the planner to the doer, and I couldn't have been happier. There were glimmers of the old Lisa shining through. Where once her bossiness would have driven us all batty, we relished in it. The day was a complete success and Lisa was so proud of her efforts; we all were.

Lisa was determined to come to Brisbane for the birth. The baby was due the week before Peter's fiftieth birthday, and the plan was to have a party on the 6th of September to celebrate both. We were so excited. Our first grandchild was on the way and our family was happy and healthy. The world was our oyster.

August 2013

Thankfully, Lisa had arrived to stay when we got the call to say Marianne had been having pains throughout the night. It was 28th August 2013. As

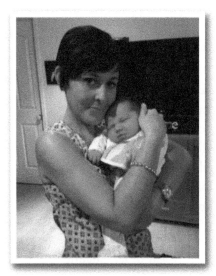

7 September 2013
Auntie / Godmother cuddles for Lisa with Ava at home at Springfield, QLD, just two days after we found out that Lisa's cancer had returned. Underneath the smiles was so much heartache.

we paced the hospital floor Lisa complained that her leggings were cutting into her a little and said she hadn't been feeling good the past few days. I was hoping she wasn't coming down with something as she had plans to go to the Gold Coast for a few days with her partner once the baby was born. They were coming back on the 5th September, the day before the party.

As the day progressed, she removed her leggings to give her some comfort. Although it helped, I could tell she was still in pain. Finally, at 5.17pm our granddaughter entered the world. She was healthy and absolutely beautiful. Our hearts were bursting.

A couple of days later, Lisa and her partner left to enjoy their few days in the sun. Although she was excited for the break and happy to know she'd be returning in a few days' time to see her gorgeous baby niece again, it was evident that she was still troubled with discomfort. She promised us that if it got any worse, she would contact her doctor in Sydney to recommend a good GP on the Gold Coast. I hoped and prayed it wouldn't come to this, not now when life was so perfect.

It's back.

Twenty-four hours later, we got a call to say Lisa had been to see a GP. The pain was now excruciating, and the doctor was taking no chances. She had sent Lisa straight for a scan. The next hour was hell. I kept telling myself that it would be okay, but in my heart of hearts I knew: that bastard was back to destroy my family. We'd been told that if the cancer returned it would be incurable.

When my phone rang, I knew what Lisa was going to say. "It's back," was all she managed before breaking down. I passed the phone to Peter to speak to her partner and then I fell apart.

The scan showed many small tumours and hotspots in Lisa's abdomen. Our cancer nightmare was back, only this time there was only one way it could end. How could the happiest time in our lives be turned into our biggest nightmare? It just wasn't fair.

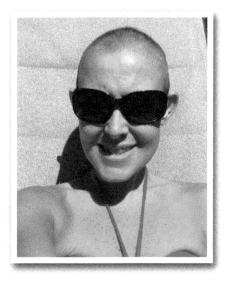

19 March 2014
Lisa sunbathing at home,
Central Coast, NSW.

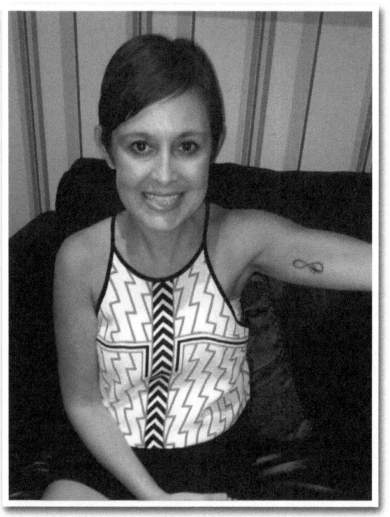

December 2014
Lisa at home showing off her new tattoo – the infinity symbol
meaning 'infinite hope'. For a long time she didn't give up hope.

The C-Word: Round Two

"A strong woman is not the one who
doesn't cry. A strong woman is the
one who cries and sheds tears for a
moment, then gets up and fights again."

~Author unknown

For the next 12 months, we went from cancer specialist to cancer specialist and trialled one treatment after another. Lisa was adamant she would not have the same chemotherapy regime she'd had previously as her quality of life would be so much less on it. She tried everything else: oral chemotherapy, numerous surgeries to cherry-pick visible tumours, steroids and many more concoctions. Each would hold off growth for a brief period and prolong Lisa's time with us. But none of the treatments were long-term solutions. In fact, many of them were trial and error. Lisa wasn't prepared to give up.

> Lisa wasn't prepared to give up.

Lisa was always googling, looking for new trials that she could take part in. She would constantly ask her oncologist if he was aware of any new treatments going on around the world. He dreaded the question as he hated telling her no. Even though he dealt with cancer patients all day every day, he showed such compassion for each of them and wanted to make them better. No matter how disheartened he felt in Lisa's appointments, he always sent her away with hope. He once told her that he had seen miracles happen before for no rhyme or reason. This was all Lisa needed to know. It was just enough to see her through to her next appointment. As long as he was still making appointments to see Lisa, she knew he was trying all he could for her.

September 2014

Lisa's oncologist told us that he had exhausted all available treatment options. The tumours were spreading throughout her abdomen but were not yet causing any problems with her organs. However, there were too many to operate on. If they operated, he said, the tumours would grow back before Lisa even had time to heal, and that's if she survived the surgery. As difficult as it was for him, he advised Lisa, pain permitting, to go and do some of the things she had always wanted to do but never had the time like travel. When Lisa pushed him for timeframes, he couldn't provide them.

Two months after this devastating news, Lisa had a major tumour bleed. Luckily, I was visiting her in New South Wales and was there when she was rushed to hospital. The medical team could not stop the bleeding and were pumping pain medication into her. Lisa's pain was excruciating. If it continued, she wouldn't make it through the night.

At one stage Lisa's eyes rolled to the back of her head. I screamed, and the medical team came rushing in. When she was finally revived, Lisa asked if she was going to die. I told her exactly what the doctor told me. "If the pain persists, they will continue to give you morphine, and with so much morphine in your body, yes, you will eventually slip away." I also told her that the family were on their way at the doctor's recommendation. Lisa immediately stopped asking for pain relief. As agonising as her pain was, her fear of dying was worse.

As a last-ditch attempt, the medical team agreed to try radiation to stop the bleed. Miraculously it worked. We were told, however, that Lisa was now terminal. We would be lucky if she was still with us at Christmas.

Upon hearing this, Lisa decided immediately that she would be moving to Queensland to be closer to us. Her partner agreed to move with her.

Peter and I also booked us all on a holiday to Hawaii, a place that Lisa had always wanted to visit. This was the best medicine ever – just what we all needed. The beautiful beaches and amazing sunsets had such a calming effect on us all. The sea was the most astonishing colour of blue, and if Lisa wasn't swimming with Ava, she was doing her next favourite thing, shopping. She shopped until she could shop no more.

Strange as it sounds, it was the most amazing family holiday we have ever had: no silly arguments and tantrums, no pressure to please others and most surprising of all, there was no pettiness from Lisa's partner. For what seemed like the first time ever, we were all on the same page, trying to squeeze a lifetime of memories into ten magical days.

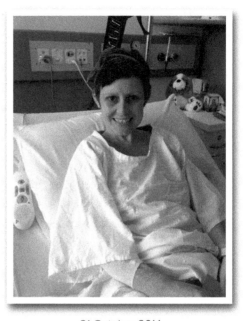

21 October 2014
Lisa at Gosford Hospital, Sydney. This hospital visit was the decider for Lisa to move to Queensland to be near her family. It was also the first time we realised that she was terminal.

On the advice of my GP, I decided to start on antidepressant medication. I needed all the help I could get to cope with our nightmare. Throughout caring for Lisa, my GP monitored my medication, increasing it if she thought it was necessary.

People often ask how we managed it. I often reply, "How could we not?"

Lisa settled well in Brisbane. She had a beautiful home sitting on the water with its own private pool and decking area. The beautiful surroundings, only 30 minutes from the family, had a positive effect on her. Because of the success of the radiation treatment, Lisa's new oncologist suggested that we continue with it as needed, that is, when the tumours were growing uncontrollably, causing pain and discomfort with the potential to result in a bleed. He also suggested trialling a new immunotherapy drug named

Keytruda, which had shown some positive results with other sarcoma patients albeit with a different type of sarcoma. We always knew we were treading uncharted waters with Lisa's disease as it was rare, with no history of effective treatment.

Once again Lisa was filled with hope. Not so much for a cure, as she knew this would be impossible, but to prolong her life. We were on an emotional rollercoaster. The highs were amazing, but we had to keep reminding ourselves that the next low could be just around the corner. We were so blessed to have found once again a medical team that looked upon Lisa as a young woman in the prime of her life and not just another statistic. Her oncologist and radiation oncologist were determined to give Lisa every opportunity possible to live the life she so courageously fought for. If they ever hesitated about further treatment, Lisa would ring them directly and browbeat them into another round of radiation.

Seven months after her move to Queensland, Lisa made the decision to end her relationship with her partner. It was not an easy decision, but it was the right one. The stress of the relationship was impacting Lisa's health and sucking the energy right out of her – energy she needed to make it through each day.

Peter and I took turns to stay with Lisa until her lease was up in November 2015, when she moved in with us. Although this was difficult for her, Lisa knew that she could no longer live in her own home. She needed full-time care, and this was the only way possible.

Peter and I also decided to sell our home right about then and buy a block of land to build our dream home on. Our friends and family worried that we were dealing with enough stress. Building the house was my idea. I had managed to convince myself that a bigger house on a better block of land would be a great investment and would help us financially when we were ready to retire. In hindsight, I always knew this was a lie. I needed a distraction, something to look forward to – a goal. I just needed something. Anything.

I felt like our bubble was getting smaller and smaller. Life was a whirlwind of medication, specialist appointments and disappointments. I was hanging on by my fingernails and began to feel immense pressure and confusion: pressure to start preparing Lisa mentally for her passing and confusion from the unknown. Rather than talking of her impending death, should I be keeping her hopes up that a cure would be found, or that we would get our much-prayed-for miracle? I asked myself continually why we were even having to think about this. Lisa should have been out there enjoying her freedom now that she was single.

There were many nights when we sat watching TV like any other family, and I would look over at Lisa. She would be reclined in her chair with four or five pre-filled syringes sitting in preparation for her next bout of pain. Her pain driver would be lying beside her pumping morphine into her as she dropped in and out of sleep. Her face was so swollen from the steroids, you would have been forgiven for thinking she was three times her actual weight. She would look so peaceful for a few minutes until the regurgitation would cause her to choke. All I could think was *Please God, if you aren't going to cure her then let her slip away.*

As desperate as I was for her to live, I was just as desperate for her pain and suffering to be over.

Sadly, around this time, we discovered that Keytruda was doing more harm than good. It was damaging Lisa's lungs and having no impact on the tumours. So the treatment was stopped immediately. The only treatment now available to Lisa was radiation, and the positive impact it had originally was now dwindling. As hard as it was to hear, to us it was just another setback. As crazy as it sounds, there comes a stage when you've been diagnosed as terminal where you become complacent. We were told so many times that there was no treatment available, or that Lisa wouldn't make it to Christmas, that we just stopping believing it.

Yes, we would shed a tear. Yes, we would feel devastated that the shot-in-the-dark treatment was not effective. But we always believed that something else would come along.

We always believed that something else would come along.

Maybe that was our way of coping.

From Desperation Came 'Terminally Fabulous'

Lisa's emotions could, understandably, be quite erratic at times. She could go from feeling so positive and determined one day to feeling so low and desperate the next. I could fully understand it. I had no control over my own emotions, and I wasn't the one with a death sentence hanging over my head. It was so hard knowing what to say and when to say it. I wanted to help but I just didn't know how. If I could have swapped places with her, I would have.

Once we had settled into our small rented property whilst waiting on our house to be built, Lisa decided to start writing a blog. Looking back, I can now see that she had wanted to start one earlier but had held off until she had ended her relationship. Her ex had been in the public eye for quite a few years, and writing a blog available to the general public would have been a no-no.

I was glad she decided to start writing. I hoped it would help her cope with what she was going through and to face what lay ahead. I also felt a little nervous about it. Lisa had never been known for her diplomacy, and I knew that in her own words 'warts and all' would mean 'warts and all'. There would be no holds barred.

Our daily challenges were about to become public.

4 July 2014
Lisa at Halekulani Hotel, Honolulu, Hawaii.
Drinks at sunset was Lisa's favourite part of
the evening. Hawaii took us to another world
where we could pretend things were normal.

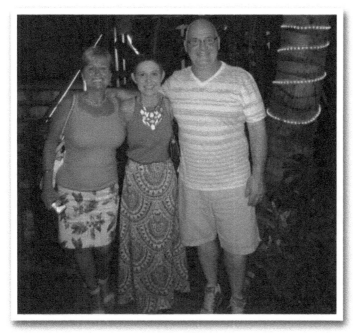

4 July 2014
Geraldine, Lisa and Peter heading out to dinner and to
watch the 4th of July fireworks in Honolulu, Hawaii.

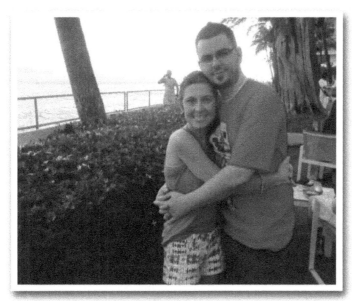

July 2014
Lisa and Steven having drinks at sunset
at Halekulani Hotel, Honolulu.

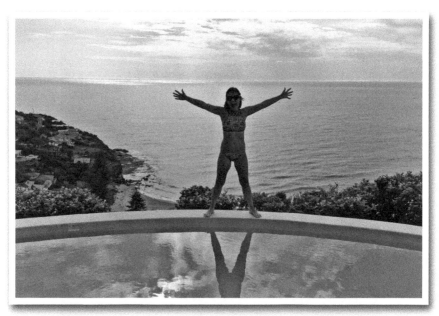

12 January 2016
Lisa Magill at Jonah's Hotel, Sydney, NSW.
"Nothing can stop me!" – Lisa

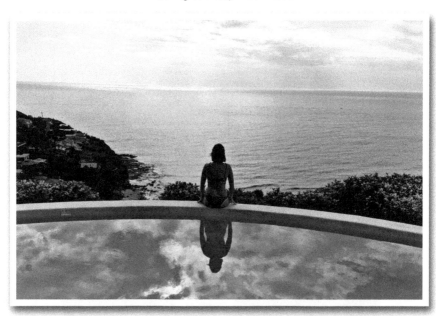

12 January 2016
Lisa at Jonah's Hotel, Sydney, NSW.
What a view! This photo was chosen for the banner
on the Terminally Fabulous website.

The Terminally Fabulous Blogs and a Mother's Reflection

About Me

1/1/2016

My name is Lisa Magill and I have been navigating the minefield that is cancer since a few months after turning 30. People have said to me for years that I should put my experiences into writing. As time progressed, I thought I had left it too late. Well, here we are nearly four years in and I've decided to attempt to blog.

What do I want you to gain from reading my blog? Well, I'm not going to say enlightenment, and I'm not going to get you to radically change your diet and start chanting at a full moon. To be quite honest the blog started out to be more about me writing it than your reading it. So if someone would happen to google cancer and inadvertently click on my link, well, that would just be a pleasant bonus. But as I develop the blog, the more I desire to reach out to those out there like me and those intrigued by my situation.

I plan on posting about the good, the bad and

> I plan on posting about the good, the bad and the ugly.

the ugly side of all things cancer, fashion, food, family — what those in the blogosphere would call a 'lifestyle blog'.

No Deal: Dexamethasone – the Drug That Deserves Its Own Blog

7/1/2016

Yeah, you know that unspoken deal I had with cancer? The one where I would allow it to live in my body and do what it's gotta do for as long as I remain me? For as long as I can remain Lisa, look like Lisa — I didn't even mind it taking my hair, TWICE — think like Lisa, be Lisa, just with a terminal disease? Well, I'm pretty certain the bitch has started to renege on our agreement (granted it was verbal and obviously there was no handshake). But up until now I was pretty certain cancer and I had an understanding, and we were preaching from the same bible.

I would say I have lost at least 70 per cent of pre-cancer Lisa. I'm almost unrecognisable. If it wasn't for regular Facebook updates and selfies, no-one would recognise me if they bumped into me in the street. Thanks to the drug dexamethasone, I'm a good 10 kilograms heavier (at least — I can't bring myself to stand on the scales); I have the lovely moon face; I have a hump growing at the base of my neck and top of my spine (yes, like the hunchback of Notre Dame); my vision is impaired; I have the hairiest face you've ever seen (seriously, I'm talking *Monkey Magic* type hairy); I have cognitive confusion and memory retention/loss issues; I'm no longer able to drive; and I am spasming in my hands, feet and back.

I am on 24-hour pain relief. I take a bloody wheelchair with me in the car everywhere I go. I have a hospital bed ordered. Yeah, an electric bed sounds cool, but for those of you who haven't had the great pleasure of sleeping more than a week on one of those things, it's like sleeping on cement after a while. Those mattresses are so bloody hard, and don't get me started on the air mattress. That thing moves all day and night, and it's noisy. I refuse to sleep on the air mattress now as it hurts my tumours.

I require a nurse to visit my home every 48 hours. I can no longer fly overseas. I can perhaps travel short interstate flights, but I need to link up with a palliative care unit wherever I go so that I can have my 48-hour nurse visits, which are sometimes every 24 hours. My palliative doctor can order me into a hospital admission if he feels I need it.

> With the loss
> of personality
> no-one can see
> outwardly what
> you've lost.

But I feel the biggest loss, other than my appearance, would be to my personality. At least with your appearance people can see that you're fighting a battle. With the loss of personality no-one can see outwardly what you've lost.

I am struggling. I am more up and down than a shopaholic who's waiting for a courier delivery. I'm more emotional than a Kim Kardashian crying emoji, and I'm one angry mofo. I just lash out like Tom Cruise in a postnatal depression debate. Things are becoming Scientology-unstable, and this is *not* acceptable to me.

Look, I've always been an opinionated and fiery type of person. If you annoy me, I'll tell you. If you upset me, you'll know it. But there's usually good reasoning behind my dislike of you: you're probably just a dick. That's fine; just don't be one around me.

I love people. I love talking to people (usually inappropriately), including random people in shops or on the street. I just love a good old chinwag and getting to know someone else's story (I get sick of my own). I like to think that over the years I've learnt to somewhat control my talent for putting my foot in it.

By the way, I have just had a little blog break as I remembered there were leftovers from dinner in the fridge in a Snap Lock® bag. I have just devoured the leftovers and turned the bag inside out and proceeded to lick the residue. Why? Because the actual food wasn't enough. I had to lick the bag! What have I become? I'll tell you what I've become: a leftovers-eating-and-licking-at-10.30pm-out-of-a-bag-because-I-couldn't-even-wait-to-put-it-on-a-plate-and-heat-it-so-I-had-to-just-devour-it-cold-out-of-the-fridge person. That's what I've become!

My mother would probably tell you otherwise, but I believe I had started to hold back a bit in recent years. I mean Mum thinks I've loved all the birthday and Christmas presents she has given me recently. Just kidding, Mum. I've loved every single one of them. I really do love you, Geraldine, and I'm so thankful for you because no-one else would put up with me. To not be in control of yourself is such a foreign experience that unless you've gone through it, I don't think you could ever fully understand it.

My biggest fear is losing my mind completely.

Cancer is hard enough by itself, never mind all the other things that come with it to basically keep me alive. I hate being all 'woe is me'. It's not the type of person I am, or is that was? I don't even know myself anymore.

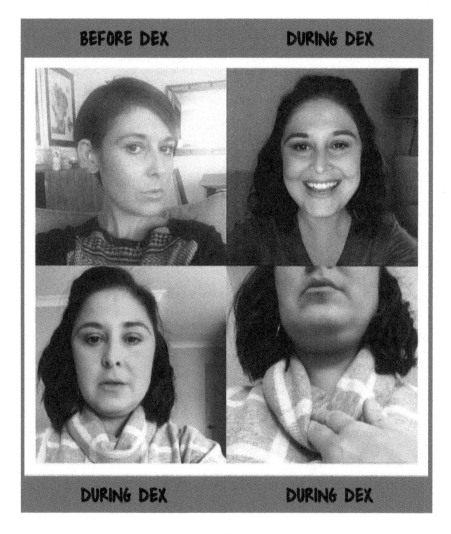

BEFORE DEX   DURING DEX

DURING DEX   DURING DEX

My biggest fear is losing my mind completely. I raised this issue the other night when I stayed in hospital. We have changed one drug, but the drug that's a non-negotiable is dexamethasone. That's the one that so far has stolen 70 per cent of me. To top it off, the doctor told me I will also continue to gain weight whilst on it. It won't just plateau one day. I will just continue to get bigger and bigger. So fabulous. I will eventually be a morbidly obese terminal cancer patient. Things are really looking up!

I look back at the photos from a year ago when I first started the drug. Luckily, I was only on it for a short time at that stage. So once I stopped it, the appearance and slow brain issues eventually subsided. It took a few months. So now I must face the fact that I will be on this drug that is the devil for good. But it is keeping my pain levels down, so it's a necessary evil.

My hope is that in six months' time, I am sitting here on my bed in my Christmas pyjamas and writing a witty, festive blog about the fact that I'm here for another Christmas, and cancer can go stuff itself. But will this drug allow me to do that?

I'm Not Done Yet

9/2/2016

As I sit here at 12.30am and listen to the rain, crying and blowing my nose, I wonder why this happens. Why do I go along for weeks and not give dying a second thought? Even when I write about it, it's as if I'm writing in the second person with a complete disconnect from me and the terminal cancer. It's as if I'm writing someone else's story. I mean, this couldn't possibly be me. I couldn't possibly be dying.

Firstly, I'm too young for this shit. Secondly, I'm still yet to achieve anything real in my life. And thirdly, I have still not taken my family to Broome or been to the Melbourne Cup as a guest in the Emirates tent. I mean, seriously, terminal cancer is meant to be for people who are in their nineties or smoked two packs a day for years. It doesn't happen to a woman who has just turned 30, drank socially, smoked a drag or two when stressed and, other than mild asthma and being coeliac (under control), has been in relatively good health all her life. No, this couldn't be about me.

Thud. There it is.

Reality.

On the 9th February 2016 at 12.25am, I remember it is me. I am the one dying. I am the one who has been finding the transition difficult. I've gone from being a woman who lived out of home, drove her own car and had a nice comfy job to this unemployed person, not allowed to drive her own car and, most difficult of all, moving back home.

It's not my parents' fault. They have done everything in their power to make the transition as easy as possible, and they care for me so much. Yet here I am, every day rolling my eyes at my mum, telling her the way she does things in 'her' household isn't right. I control who can come and who can go. It depends on whether they have a runny nose (which could be a cold that can turn into big infections or a virus that could lead to my death from a compromised immune system) or if I'm in the mood mentally for it or not. I should be trying to fit in and we should all be trying to work together. A bit my way, a bit Mum's way. Let's be serious; with two women in the house, there's no room left for Dad to have anything his way.

So tonight, as I looked at myself in the mirror about to brush my teeth – *shit, that reminds me I didn't get around to brushing my teeth* – I saw the person in the reflection who is dying, and it is me. And I am making my mum's life especially difficult. She has to deal with knowing that her daughter could die at any moment. She could walk into my room tomorrow and find me lifeless. We could be watching TV tomorrow night and I have a massive tumour bleed and that's it. All over red rover.

So why does my stupid mouth insist on speaking before it starts thinking? Because I have been so used to running my own race, house-wise I mean. Like silly things: toilet roll over or under (over of course) and glasses and cups, rim up or rim down (up of course, for no reason). The list of stupid and insignificant things that I make nagging comments on is endless. Meanwhile, my mum is run ragged mentally, trying to not only get on top of the fact that her daughter is expiring in front of her eyes, but also that her daughter is just not happy with anything she does. And the truth is, Mum does everything 100 per cent right. It's just 100 per cent right her way, and that's what I have to realise. Not only did I run my own race, so did my mum.

So, I had this overwhelming need to hug my mum. I don't know if it's because I'm scared for some reason that I might not wake up tomorrow. I mean, I have no more of a reason today than I did yesterday to think I'm going to die in my sleep tonight. And I didn't even think about it last night. So, like I said in my opening sentence to this blog, why tonight other than I think I needed a good kick up the arse to realise that my mum does nothing but try to please me from morning until night?

> I've always loved lying in bed at night listening to the rain dancing on the roof.

One thing I do know is it's raining. I've always loved lying in bed at night listening to the rain dancing on the roof.

So, although I've realised again (as I do every few weeks) that, yes, I am writing about myself, not some 95-year-old, smoking and drinking a glass of whiskey, I remember why I've fought so hard to keep on living:

- I'm not done learning.
- I'm not done loving.
- And I'm not done laughing.

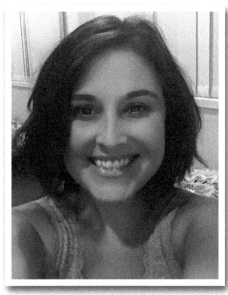

25 February 2016
Lisa at home in Springfield Lakes, QLD. She wasn't going to give up!

I just hope whoever or whatever has kept me going this long realises that I'm not ready to go. Not just yet.

Familiarity Breeds Contempt

29/02/2016

"But you look so well!"

I hear this numerous times a day, but actually I am not well. I have terminal cancer. For every smiling selfie you see of me on Facebook or Instagram there is an equally unattractive reality of shooting up hydromorphine hourly to keep on top of pain.

I am a 34-year-old woman who has had to recently move back in with her parents (whom I haven't lived with since I was 19) as I require 24-hour care (well, prefer to call it 'surveillance') as I can have a tumour bleed at any time and need immediate hospitalisation. During some of these bleeds I cannot breathe. I am curled up in a ball with pain so intense that I can't speak. So as you can imagine, calling an ambulance can become difficult.

For those of you who are lucky enough to still have a mum and/or dad in their lives, and even luckier to have had your relationship reach a point that you are now friends with your parents (you no longer put up with them so you'll be allowed to stay out past curfew and you actively choose to go out to dinner with them and even pay for it) you have come full circle. It's a wonderful stage in life. Prior to moving back in with my parents, we had obtained parent-child perfection. We were the family people envied for our closeness. Cancer brought us even closer. We were grateful for every extra moment we got to spend together. Fast forward from November last year to now, and I am titling a blog post 'Familiarity Breeds Contempt'!

Don't get me wrong. My parents and I get along great; it's just full-on! Mum is my 24-hour carer (unpaid) and we spend most of those hours together. Our problem is that we are too similar. We are both highly sensitive and are always trying to please everybody. And that is simply impossible.

It also doesn't help that I am impossible to live with at the best of times,

40

never mind throwing terminal cancer and a myriad of opioids into my already highly-developed OCD mix. Throw in an eye-rolling problem too. Only today Mum asked if I could use the eye roll a little more sparingly. Well, actually, no. No, I can't. Stupid behaviour has a direct correlation between my brain and my optic nerve. If you continue to behave stupidly, I will continue to eye-roll. Alter your behaviour and I will alter mine accordingly. Well, that's the conversation I had in my head. I, of course, agreed to be more mindful of my eye rolling in the future. There you have a ticking time bomb. Or do you?

We have acknowledged the stress my moving in has put on our relationship and on my parents' relationship. When do they ever get a chance to debrief and destress? I am always around.

Just like Mum forgot how annoying my eye rolls can be, I forgot how annoying my dad can be with his constant finger tapping and background noise. He just simply cannot 'be'. He has to be making some sort of noise. He's currently banging around in the kitchen as I type.

> Familiarity has more pros than cons.

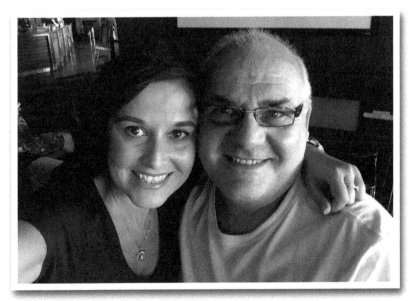

31 October 2015
Lisa and her dad Peter Magill at Boardwalk Tavern, Hope Island, QLD.

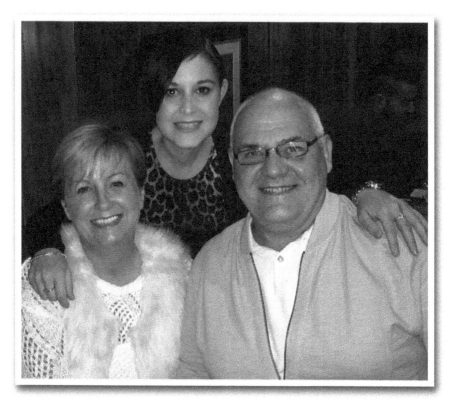

30 July 2015
Geraldine, Lisa and Peter out to dinner in Hobart, TAS.

So for now, as we reintroduce each other to our annoying habits and try to realign our behaviour so that we can make living with each other somewhat bearable again, I just want you to remember that the familiar isn't always bad. In fact, familiarity has more pros than cons. It's just hard to think of the pros while my dad bangs his empty cereal bowl and teaspoon in the sink as he has done since before the dawn of time. (He has always eaten his cereal with a teaspoon.) He leaves a bowl filled with water and his teaspoon sitting in the sink every morning when I wake up, just as it was when I was a kid. It's familiarity, and it makes me smile.

I'd love to read this and say that Lisa's late-night recollection of how difficult things were then was completely incorrect. Unfortunately, it's not.

Peter and I had longed for Lisa to move home. We wanted to take care of her, to be there for her and, most of all, to show her how much we loved her. Whatever time she had left, we wanted to spend it with her. But it was always going to be challenging. Between pain meds, steroids, strong personalities and one medical disappointment after another, things were never going to be easy.

Lisa had to eat a gluten-free diet. I understood what was involved with cooking gluten-free meals, but cooking dinner became my worst nightmare. Lisa would supervise my every move. I would pray that she would fall asleep before I started prepping, but it was like she had bionic ears. As soon as I'd walk into the kitchen, she was there watching my every move and shooting orders. Dinner time often ended in tears – usually mine.

Getting ready to go to appointments was just as challenging. Lisa would quite often feel stressed prior to seeing her medical team, which is understandable. Therefore, getting out the door was a major stress. She would designate herself so much time for every task: shower, hair, make-up, medication and so on. She would set the alarm on her phone to ensure she kept to the designated times. Quite often those timings would go out the window for one reason or another, and it would all go downhill from there. We usually arrived at appointments frazzled.

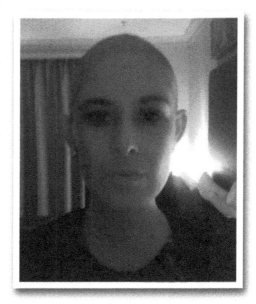

29 February 2016

That being said, by the time I went to bed at night I would force myself to forget (or bury) what had happened during the day – easier said than done. I knew Lisa didn't mean a lot of what she said, but it hurt. I felt there was nothing I could do right, and the mental strain started to wear me down. I never doubted my love for Lisa, but I often doubted my ability to care for her as she wanted to be cared for. As hard as Lisa tried, she couldn't control her mood swings and I was walking on eggshells.

I was fully aware that Peter was the familiarity and I was the contempt. Seeing it in Lisa's blog hurt. I asked her to remove it, but she refused. However, the more I thought about it the more I agreed with her. This was reality. As the mum and carer, I was the one constantly open to criticism. Peter and I could do the exact same thing in the exact same way, but mine was never done right.

As much as I struggled with it, I wouldn't have traded places with anyone. I needed to be there. I wanted to be there.

Who Cares What You Look Like? You're Alive

05/03/2016

I am currently at war with my own body, and I'm not just talking about the cancer. I'm talking about my appearance.

As mentioned in my previous blog about my chipmunk, marshmallow-cheeked Lara-Flynn-Boyle-bloated-hairy-as-Wolverine face, my body has also decided to join the bloating party. And it seems it was BYOC as well (bring your own cellulite).

Since beginning the immunotherapy Keytruda in November (treatment via infusion through a port in my chest once every three weeks), I have gained about 8 kilos (about 17.5 pounds or 1.25 stone). "Eight kilos," you say. "That's not much!" Well, on a 4-foot 11-inch woman, an 8-kilo weight gain is very noticeable. In fact, 2 kilos are very noticeable. It's from a combination of the drug Dexamethasone (a steroid) as well as other drugs I'm prescribed ... Plus eating ... My appetite is insatiable 24 hours a day, which is a drug side effect.

Basically, I'm retaining bucketloads of fluid that they call 'disproportionate bloating'. So it can make you look lopsided or fatter on one side of your face, stomach and limbs than the other. This has happened with my under-the-chin fat. Yes, I now have under-the-chin fat.

I am frantically eating my parents out of house and home. I eat a loaf of bread a day (gluten free as I'm coeliac — we'll get to that in another blog) and pasta. Plus I drink Coke by the bucketloads. (A year ago, you could count on two hands the amount of Coke I would have drank in a one-year period). I eat red cloud lollies, gluten-free Special K, ham, chicken, chips, cheese ... you name it. If it's not healthy I am eating it.

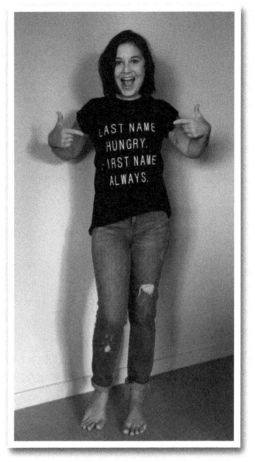

8 January 2016
Lisa — Last name Hungry, First name Always

My belly is bloated to the point where the bellies of my friends, who are posting their seven-month pregnancy belly photos on Facebook, are actually smaller than mine. It is rock hard. I also have hard lumps all over my stomach from injecting drugs. They look very attractive, like ping pong balls under the skin. It basically looks like an exaggerated cartoon form of cellulite on my stomach. I can't wear form-fitting clothes as they push on my tumours and cause me pain.

My legs are bruised, bloated and lumpy, also from the drugs I inject. As I've mentioned before people say, "Who cares? You've got cancer and you're still here fighting it. Who cares if you've gained weight or have a hairy face?"

45

I'll tell you who cares about weight gain and appearance: Every single woman that's ever been born, that's who!

Just because a person gets cancer does not mean that they automatically become this self-loving, enlightened individual. Why should cancer make me behave like any less of who I was before? Because I am sick, am I meant to leave the 'old' me behind and embrace the 'new' me like some long-lost relative? What makes people think that all we are is our cancer?

> We are not just our cancer.

We are not just our cancer. We are wives, girlfriends, mothers, entrepreneurs, best friends and, most of all, we are still WOMEN!!!!!

So do me a favour. If you have a friend that has cancer and they are going through (or recovering from) treatment and are bald, have no eyelashes and eyebrows, have bad acne, skin discolouration, cold sores, bloating, are fat and the list goes on, don't tell them, "You're lucky to be alive. Who cares what you look like?" Instead empathise with them. Obviously, you're not going to say "Yeah, you do kinda look like a bloated hairy-in-all-the-wrong-places alien with bad skin, tally ho!" Perhaps tell them you could never begin to imagine how they feel, so you're not even going to try.

Your friend has just been through, or is going through, one of the most harrowing experiences any human being should ever have to endure. Tell them you love them and that you are there for them no matter what. If they want to spend an hour bitching and moaning about how ugly they feel, just be there. Listen and don't judge. Certainly, don't rationalise. There is no rationale when it comes to cancer.

Just let us vent and hate the world and ourselves for a minute. Then as any good friend would, go to the kitchen and get the tub of ice-cream out and two spoons. The post-cancer diet, like all diets, can always start tomorrow.

Lisa was always honest about how she felt about her everchanging face and body. She was a beautiful girl in the prime of her life when cancer stuck.

Her hair, make-up and clothes had to be perfect before she would leave the house. It was not unusual for Lisa to spend two hours getting ready. In fact, it was a running joke in our house.

I would sit in Lisa's appointments and cringe when Dexamethasone was mentioned. She absolutely hated the damage it did to her face, body and mind. Dexi, as we nicknamed it, took away one of the very few things she felt she had control of: her looks. She knew toxic drugs like chemo and

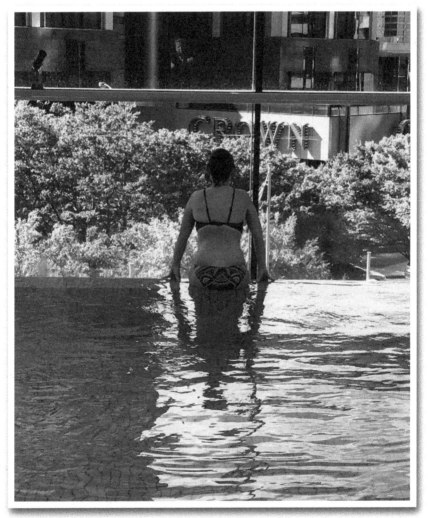

15 March 2016
Lisa having a dip in the pool at the Crown Hotel, Melbourne, VIC.

radiation did irreparable damage to her insides, but she could block them out. She didn't have to look at them every day.

To us she remained beautiful throughout. But to Lisa it was heartbreaking.

A Radiating Week in More Ways Than One

19/03/2016

Radiate: (of light or heat) emitted in the form of rays or waves, (person) clearly emanate a strong feeling or quality through their expression or bearing.

This week has been exactly that. It radiated life, laughter, love, fun, pain and more. I had a visit from a wonderful overseas friend who has beamed a ray of light into my life like no other. I spent the day doing something with her, her best friend, my friend and my mum that I have never done in my life before, and I will most likely never do again. That day was full on, and at the end of it I was in a decent amount of pain. But you just keep injecting yourself with your pain meds and soldier on.

My pain unfortunately has been getting increasingly worse. I have used more pain medication in the last two months than I have in the last four years of having cancer. Our fears were confirmed when I ended up in hospital and got scanned. The results showed that all my tumours are growing and the immunotherapy that we were paying thousands of dollars every three weeks for did not work.

> There is no way I am going to let this thing just take me down without a fight.

So what now? Do I lie down and let this bastard take me? Or do I look at other options?

Hell yes. I look at other options.

There is no way I am going to let this thing just take me down without a fight. I have to admit I did have a moment (it was fleeting) where I had a cry and a whinge and thought, *How much more of this can one person take?* We just keep

48

throwing everything at this cancer and it laughs in our faces. It takes our money, our time, my health.

I am hoping I will be afforded the opportunity to say, "That's enough now. I've done all that I can possibly do and that's enough". But the reality is I will most likely have a massive tumour bleed, bleed out and die within minutes. There will most likely not be the need for a stay-at-home nurse like you see in the movies (that does happen though) or a bedside vigil where I get to speak wonderful words of wisdom to each of my loved ones. That's why I tell them every day what I want them to know, both good and bad.

This week also had radiotherapy! Radiotherapy uses radiation, such as X-rays, gamma rays, electron beams or protons, to kill or damage cancer cells and stop them from growing and multiplying. It is a localised treatment, which means it generally only affects the part of the body where the radiation is directed. But because my disease is so widespread and near so many vital organs, directing the rays can be difficult. You do not want them to hit your liver, kidneys or other vital organs!

To avoid this, you have a planning scan a few days prior to treatment where the radiation therapists measure the precise spots that need to be radiated. This involves lying on a CT machine practically naked. A couple of women move you around to align your body with treatment areas and then tattoo small dots on your body as markers for when you

> They stand there and talk around me like a piece of meat ready to be diced and sliced.

have your radiation. It's all done using lines and angles and measurements. Very clinical. They use terms like 'centigray' (the measurement of the amount of radiation absorbed by the patient's body), 'fractionation' (dividing total dose of radiation into smaller doses to try and save as much healthy tissue as possible) and 'dosimetrist' (the person who plans the radiation dose). Basically, I hear the teacher from Charlie Brown's *Peanuts* comic as they stand there and talk around me like a piece of meat ready to be diced and sliced into sections.

Then, on treatment day, you lie on a cold, hard steel slab for around 40 minutes with your hands raised above your head in a freezing treatment room. You have to lie perfectly still while panels rotate around your body emitting a laser-type treatment. No itchy nose scratching, no sneezing, no movement whatsoever. Try lying perfectly still for over 40 minutes. Not to mention the fact that lying down in any normal circumstance is painful for me because my tumours are suffocating my organs and pinching nerves.

Whilst they are basically invisibly burning away at your tumour tissue (and hopefully not your healthy tissue), a stream of 'soothing music' is being played over a sound system. One of the appropriately chosen songs last night was *Toxic* by Britney Spears. I mean, seriously people, have we cancer patients not had enough toxicity pumped through our veins already that you have to remind us that we're toxic whilst receiving treatment? I mean I love a good Britney beat, but a little bit of sensitivity wouldn't go astray. You may as well play bloody *Wind Beneath My Wings* or *Tears in Heaven*!

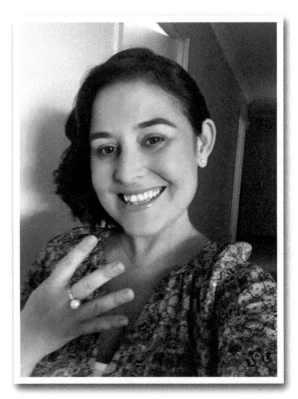

29 March 2016
Lisa at home in Springfield Lakes, QLD, after her fourth session of radiation.

I am having four sessions at this point. As I type in bed I have, just hours ago, completed my first of this round and am already dealing with the lovely side effects. I had numerous spots radiated in my abdomen, and I also had the two golf-ball-sized pelvic tumours targeted. Now I feel nauseated. I've been up most of the night vomiting. My stomach is cramping, and I've been hobbling (to say running would be a wee bit of an exaggeration) to the toilet with the loose bowels the nurses mentioned may happen. My bladder is sore, and I've taken numerous hydromorphone injections to try and get on top of the pain.

And I'm sitting here typing a bloody blog. Am I mad in the head or what?

One thing that I don't know to laugh or cry about is the baby monitor currently sitting on my bedside table, which monitored me last night in case pain got too much and I couldn't let Mum and Dad know. I've gone from *Playboy Babes* to baby monitors all in the space of 24 hours. I swear someone up there is having a good old laugh right now.

I will keep you updated on the progress of my radiotherapy and let you know if anything interesting happens.

I always describe the cancer journey as a never-ending rollercoaster ride. There were so many highs and lows, and this blog was a perfect example.

During one of our bucket list experiences, we were staying at the Versace Hotel on the Gold Coast with some girlfriends. We were aware that Kendra Wilkinson was also staying there as she had been filming a UK TV show locally with a large group of celebrities. I was talking to Kendra's dad at the hotel reception desk and happened (on purpose) to mention Lisa's love for Kendra and the reason we were at the hotel. He was truly lovely and told me he would arrange for Kendra to meet with Lisa. True to his word we had a call to our suite not long after, asking us to come up to Kendra's room as she was being interviewed. Once finished she wanted to spend the day with us.

Lisa had an amazing day. Kendra treated Lisa as though she was a lifelong friend and constantly praised her strength and determination. Even with distance between them, Lisa and Kendra remained the best of friends. The visit Lisa mentions in her blog was with Kendra and her best friend Jess, Lisa, me and Lisa's friend Aleana. We spent the day filming with them in Melbourne for Kendra's show *Kendra on Top*. Lisa was a natural and chatted away as though the camera wasn't even there. The girls were like long-lost family and truly made Lisa the star of the show. She had the time of her life and I couldn't have been prouder (and more thankful).

After that high of our rollercoaster ride came the low. From overdoing it the tumours had swollen somewhat and Lisa's pain levels were excruciating. No amount of morphine could bring them under control, and so began another round of radiation when we returned to Brisbane. Although there

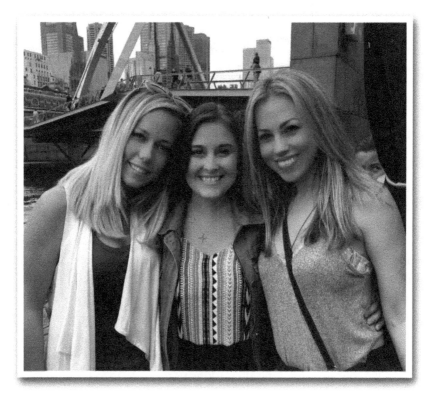

14 March 2016
Lisa having drinks with Kendra Wilkinson and Jessica Hall at Southbank, Melbourne, VIC, after filming an episode of *Kendra On Top*. Kendra and Lisa built a strong friendship after one brief encounter. Kendra and Jess remain family friends.

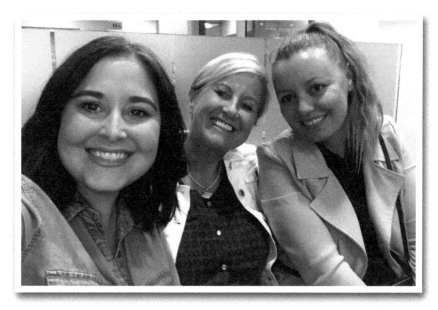

8 September 2016
Lisa, Geraldine and Aleana McGuiness at Greenslopes Private
Hospital. Another hospital appointment with a bestie's support.

14 March 2016
Lisa at Richmond Hospital,
Melbourne, VIC. After meeting
Kendra and Jess and a full day
of filming, Lisa's pain went above
manageable levels, so a short
visit to hospital was needed to
get things back under control.

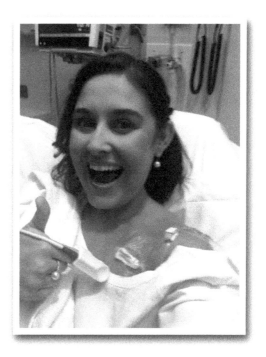

was a price to pay for living life like any other 34-year-old, Lisa never had any regrets. Along with the fear, pain and misery there had to be days full of fun and excitement.

A Mother-Daughter Perspective

21/03/2016

"Hello, it's back." – three words no mother of a child that's had cancer ever wants to hear.

The 5th of September 2013 was the day my mum received a phone from me from my car in a random carpark, at a random imaging centre on the Gold Coast. It was eight days after the birth of her first grandchild and one day before my dad's 50th birthday and birthday party. Timing is never good when it comes to this, but the timing really couldn't have been much worse for any of us.

I had been experiencing horrendous pain in the lead-up to the birth of my niece Ava. On the day of the birth I'd had to remove my leggings as they felt like they were strangling my stomach and bladder. Days after, I was in the car with my brother and going over speed humps in a carpark and asking him, "Are these speed humps not hurting your stomach, driving over them?" I then went away for a couple of days with my then-partner to the Gold Coast. He went to the chemist across from the hotel for me, and I collapsed in a ball of pain in the hotel room. The pain only lasted minutes, but it was bad.

When my partner returned, he insisted that I visit a doctor – he'd been insisting the entire week – so I relented. We rang around, found a doctor and he got me in for an ultrasound straight away. The doctor had actually put my mind at ease as he thought it was perhaps a surgical hernia. He didn't think it felt like a tumour. I even rang my mum and told her the doctor's thoughts to allay her fears.

As I was lying there, I noticed the ultrasound technician was taking a rather long time to find what should be as straightforward as a hernia. She added more gel and the field of the ultrasound started to get bigger. Certain parts

54

that she was pressing on caused me to recoil in pain, and she apologised. Then I saw it, that look, the look I'd seen before. The I-know-what-this-is-but-I'm-not-allowed-to-tell-you-what-it-is-that's-up-to-your-doctor look. The I'd-hate-to-be-you look. The technician excused herself and came back in with a doctor. On this occasion they just came out and said it. They afforded me the dignity of letting me know that my cancer was back before telling the Gold Coast doctor, subsequently avoiding the stress of waiting 24 hours to hear from him.

"How did you feel when you found out it was back?"

This is a question I've asked a few friends and family to answer for me for the blog, so I suppose I should answer it first. I felt pain – immense pain – a pounding in my chest, a ringing in my ears, a lump the size of Gibraltar in my throat. Everything was just white noise. 'Incurable' was being repeated in my head because that's what my oncologist had said in my initial treatment. "If it comes back, you're incurable." My mind didn't even go into survival mode, like it normally would. It went into fear mode, something I'm not used to.

I make plans. I make plans in case plans about plans about plans fail. There is always a back-up plan. Suddenly I thought, *Well, not now. I have no control over this. I cannot change it. Death, funerals. What will my loved ones do? I'm not going to see Ava go to school, get married.* Thoughts just flooded me – overwhelming thoughts of death and how much longer I have. There is no way to describe how a person truly feels upon hearing this news. It's an out-of-body experience, a mind-numbing 'Is-this-really-happening?' experience.

I came out crying, so my partner surmised it was back, and then he started crying. Reception bulk billed the scan (paid by the government), so I didn't need to worry about that on top of everything else. I rang my doctor in Sydney to let them know as they were closing in minutes, so I could organise an action plan. Then there I was, sitting in the carpark on the other end of the phone call that I never wanted to have to make.

It's not all about me. Cancer affects everyone around you.

For this blog I asked my mum to tell me her experience, in her own words, in her own way. I want this blog to give different perspectives because, at the end of the day, it's not all about me. Cancer affects everyone around you. I hope her perspective may help someone else's mum or dad out there, who may be at the receiving end of that telephone call or may have already received it.

Mum's words:

Thinking back to how I originally felt when Lisa was diagnosed with terminal cancer, my first reaction was to go into grieving mode.

I was haunted by thoughts of death and many questions went through my mind: What did Lisa want at the end? How were we going to bury our own daughter? How would our life be without our daughter? What would we answer when people asked how many children we had? Why Lisa and why not me, and how in God's name were we going to get through this?

Sleep was impossible as my mind wouldn't let me rest. My heart was so sore, and my days were blurred. There were days when the treatment was

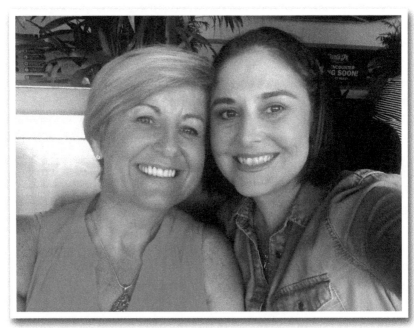

13 March 2016
Geraldine and Lisa at Brisbane Airport on the way to Melbourne.

so harsh that I just wanted the suffering to end. But then I'd remind myself that the only way this could happen was death. I'd arrive at the hospital and be numb with fear, worrying about what lay ahead.

Many times, I sat in the hospital treatment room feeling like an observer, looking in on a situation that couldn't be real. Surgeries were especially tough for me. As Lisa was wheeled away I would go weak at the knees until she returned to her room.

One morning I woke up with the realisation that I was living life as if Lisa had already passed. I was posting all these positive quotes filled with hope on Facebook, but they were for Lisa's benefit. I didn't truly believe them. I decided there and then that my head was going to protect my heart. I would make the most of the good days and do my best to support Lisa on the bad days. This has worked well for me. It keeps me strong and focused on what's going on and enables me to get through the hardest days.

At times, I feel I must come across as hard to others and without feeling. This couldn't be further from the truth. Weekly counselling sessions keep me grounded but also allow me time to break down and face reality whilst giving me the strength to go care for Lisa the best way I can. —Geraldine

I was so glad when Lisa asked me to write how I felt when her cancer returned. I was highly emotional but thankful. I wanted her followers, who had come to love and support her, to know how I truly felt as a mother. Not as the person that could stuff up a gluten-free meal or aggravate Lisa by my calm approach to being at appointments on time, but as a mum whose heart was breaking just at the thought of losing her only daughter.

I wanted people to understand how I felt, and just for one moment to know what I was going through.

When Lisa was originally diagnosed, we were heartbroken but naïve. We had no idea what lay ahead, though we knew it would be extremely difficult. Lisa's cancer returning when it did was unfathomable. I remember hanging up from Lisa's call and asking God what the F@#$ He thought

He was doing. How could He do this to our family? Had He not made us suffer enough? Did we look too happy? I just couldn't get my head around it. I was dying inside.

Once again, our world was falling apart and there was nothing we could do. This time it was the exact opposite of the first. We knew exactly what lay ahead and it terrified us beyond belief.

That One Question that Makes Me Feel Inadequate...

25/03/2016

Just a warning relating to this blog: It is slightly different to my normal blog style. In this one I am airing a grievance that has just annoyed me again this evening. So I felt I had to write about it. I've said from the start that this blog will be warts and all. Enjoy x

A question I often get asked by people after telling them I have terminal cancer is a question I think is common to female cancer patients in their thirties. It's "Do you have kids?" When I respond no, they often say something along the lines of "Aw, it's probably a good thing. At least you don't have to worry about that". Or I've been told it's a blessing as I wouldn't need that extra stress of worrying about their wellbeing. It's also accompanied by a sort of disappointed look, a head tilt and a change in tone of voice, like a gentle soothing 'there-there' voice.

When I am asked that question, I get a knot in my stomach. I feel somewhat unworthy, like I haven't achieved the right things in life. I feel like the woman who has three children in the bed next to me with terminal cancer would deserve the *Better Homes & Gardens* renovation more than me because she will be leaving a husband and children behind. I'll be leaving a Chanel handbag and a few pairs of Louboutins. Who cares about my parents losing a child or my loved ones losing me? They don't matter.

The truth of the matter is that cancer took away that option. My treatments have put me into a menopausal state three times now. The closest I get to a tampon these days is Aisle 12 at Woollies.

This got me thinking that this must be a common thing for all women out there. Yeah, I'm talking to you, the ones who are single. The ones in long-term relationships who still haven't got a ring on; the ones in a relationship who have tried desperately to fall pregnant and haven't, or sadly have and lost. You would definitely get the head tilt.

What is it about us human beings that we feel we have the right to judge others on their marital, parental and even employment status? I am a 34-year-old unmarried, unemployed, childless woman. I have really broken the glass ceiling. Those judgmental Judies out there must love it when they start firing their questions at me. I am the 'well-things-could-be-worse-I-could-be-Lisa' person.

Why should we be made to feel like subpar human beings? So what if we didn't get married? Maybe I'm infertile. Did you ever think about that when you asked that question? I have many friends who have struggled terribly with falling pregnant, and I feel horrible for them when people ask about kids. I know people aren't asking these questions out of malice. It's in general interest and often care. I just think people need to gauge their audience better. Maybe think before you ask.

Have you ever stopped and thought that maybe, just maybe, it's an actual lifestyle choice? Maybe my 34-year-old friend loves being single, going out to a club, dancing all night and crawling into bed at 6am. And she might be crawling into bed with someone else that she may or may not have just met in the kebab shop on the way home. (This is purely fictional, so for my single friends out there, I am not talking about you.) Have you ever stopped to think that your friends that have been married for 15 years, with two dogs called Will and Grace and a parakeet named Poopsy, have chosen not to procreate? Maybe they'd prefer to put potential school fees into that European trip they're doing first-class-return next August.

There are so many different types of people out there with different relationships and different ideals. No person should ever be made to feel less worthy than the next just because they haven't achieved what society believes is the norm. We're in the era of the new norm. I mean, seriously, when Bruce Jenner was winning gold in the Decathlon in 1976, I really don't believe anyone would have envisaged that some 40 years later she'd be called Caitlyn and be winning *Glamour* magazine's Woman of the Year. Surely if Caitlyn Jenner can be crowned Woman of the year (go girl!), we can accept that a woman in her thirties has not procreated.

Keep living YOUR life.

So to all of you out there that don't fit snugly into the box that is 'normality', I salute you. Keep living YOUR life. Yes, that's right, YOUR life. The next time someone asks me that question, I don't think I'll feel the knot in my stomach like I used to. I think I'll just embrace it and accept that it is really a perfectly reasonable question. It's just the pity parade that comes with it doesn't sit well with me. So I'll just ignore that part and maybe ask them if they prefer it on top or on the bottom.

On that note, I'm off to bed. 2am has rolled around quickly.

Re-reading the last blog was extremely difficult for me. I can see how I sometimes fell into the category of people that Lisa talks about who say, "You're alive, aren't you?" except not quite in the same way. I knew there were terrible after-effects that came with chemo. I knew that Lisa would never have children. I knew she loved her hair and would lose it. But I also knew that having treatment was going to give Lisa more time. All I would allow myself to focus on was Lisa and how I could help her. My head and heart couldn't cope with any more.

Now, in hindsight, I can't help but hurt at the thought of Lisa never having her own child, and Peter and I not having a grandchild from Lisa. And I hate the fact that Ava won't have a cousin living nearby who will eventually become her best friend. I hate that cancer had Lisa racked with pain for the last four years of her life. But mostly I hate that she didn't get to experience life as a normal 34-year-old, looking forward to what lay ahead of her and achieving the goals she'd set for herself.

I just wanted her to live a normal healthy, happy life. I just wanted her to live.

60

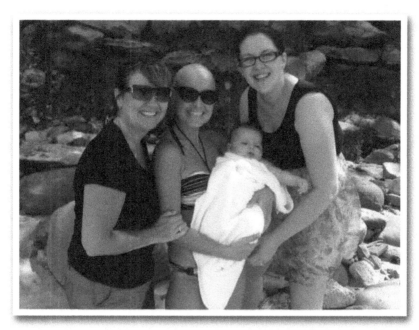

5 December 2013
Geraldine, Lisa, Ava and Marianne on the Central
Coast, NSW, for Ava's first swim with Lisa.

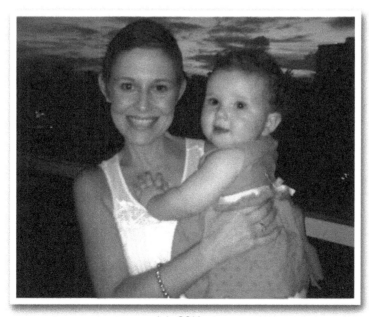

July 2014
Lisa and Ava on the hotel balcony in Honolulu enjoying cuddles at sunset.

Chemo: To Vomit or Not to Vomit?

28/03/2016

...It's Not Really an Option, More of a Necessity

This is a long one people. Better put the kettle on.

A large part of any cancer patient's life is treatment. When you're first diagnosed, the first question you will most likely ask is: "Am I going to die?" I'd say the second would be: "Ok, so where to from here? What treatment? Am I going to have to have chemo?" Well, that's what my questions were. Actually, if I'm completely honest, after "Am I going to die?" (the first time I was told I had cancer), my next question was "Am I going to lose my hair?"

My hair was my crowning glory. From the age of 15, I had long, lusciously-thick dark brown hair. Yes, it may have been a chemical reproduction for a few years near the end there – I started to go grey at 18 – but the hair itself was mine. I was never the tall girl, the thin girl or the hot girl. I was always the short girl with long hair. The long hair was my thing. It was at that stage in my life that I believed my hair to be my only redeeming feature looks-wise.

So my first thought was *Am I going to lose it?* Now I don't know if this is something all oncologists say, but three different oncologists have told me during different chemotherapy treatments that there is a 'chance' I may lose my hair. None of them ever really confirmed it for me, which in my opinion is way worse.

Just tell me. Don't give me this false hope that I may fall in the one-and-a-half per centile bracket of people who don't lose their hair using a particular chemo. Of course, the first thing we do when we walk out of that consultation is google the drug and find it doesn't just say 'hair thinning' but 'hair loss'! So just afford us the decency and at least say you're most likely going to lose your hair. Because this false hope crap is pointless. Maybe other oncologists are more straightforward with their patients, but mine certainly weren't when it came to treatment symptoms.

When it comes to treatment, for some reason I feel I've gotten off lightly. I hear of these people who are on chemo for a year and do 100 radiotherapy sessions, and I think I've been pretty lucky.

My first chemotherapy was a combination of two chemo drugs called doxorubicin and ifosfamide. I would go into the chemo day ward, where a nurse (dressed up like she was in an Ebola quarantine ward) would cannulate me and hook me up to the toxic 'life saver'. Then I'd sit for eight hours having this thick red liquid, followed by a clear one, pumped into my veins. I'd then be wheel-chaired, usually by this stage with a sick bag in hand, vomiting, to the cancer ward at St Vincent's in Sydney.

I remember the first time I went into the ward. There were four beds in each room. A woman in the bed next to me looked like she was minutes away from passing: skeletal-skinny, ghostly pale and just lying there in a vegetative state. This boosted my morale right up! I then stayed in the hospital for 72 hours, receiving chemotherapy for the first 48. (By the way the woman on death's doorstep in the bed next to me was up and about the next day like a sprightly rabbit.) Then I was monitored to make sure my liver and kidneys wouldn't fail for the next 24 hours and went home.

The first three days in hospital after treatment weren't really the worst. There was a bit of vomiting, a heavy head and a lot of sleeping. But it was the days after, for about a week or two, that were hardest. I had constant nausea, an indescribable tiredness, a constant stale taste in my mouth, mouth ulcers, body and bone aches from a needle they gave me to make my white cells grow back faster, bloating, constipation, diarrhoea, weight gain or weight loss – I gained 7 kilos during my first chemo – rashes, loss of taste and depression. Plus my nails began to rot away in front of my eyes.

What a lot of people don't know is that when you start to lose your hair, it actually hurts. Your scalp aches at every hair cuticle. If you lie down on a pillow, your head pounds and the weight of your hair pulling on the cuticle is sheer agony. As soon as my hair started to come out in clumps, I cut it and shaved it off. It was the best decision I ever made because as soon as I shaved it, the headaches and pain went. So I highly recommend not putting up with it; just get rid of it. Honestly, you'll thank me in the long run.

> When you start to lose your hair, it actually hurts.

By the third cycle of treatment, if your chemo does cause hair loss (not all chemo does), you will most likely lose ALL of your hair. Yes, down there, front, back and sides, eyelashes and eyebrows. That last one is the worst as it gives you that lovely 'alienesque' look. People look at you and can't quite figure out what doesn't look right. The only place I didn't lose hair was on my arms – the one place I would have loved. It did turn white though.

I've described before that chemo is like having the worst hangover you could ever imagine, every day for nearly three weeks, combined with going on the amusement park ride, the Gravitron. You know, the circular one where you stand with your back to the wall and the ride spins endlessly (or that's how it feels). When you get off you don't know if you want to be sick or end your life. These two things combined times 1000, and there you have an apt description of chemo side effects. Then when you finally start to feel almost human again, you have to skull another ten bottles of tequila, hop back on the Gravitron and the carrousel of chemo side effects begin again.

You are also classed as cytotoxic when you're on chemotherapy, meaning if you vomit you are effectively spewing toxic sewage harmful to anyone who comes in contact with it. It needs to be cleaned up with special gloves and disposed of in a special bag, so you don't give someone toxic poisoning.

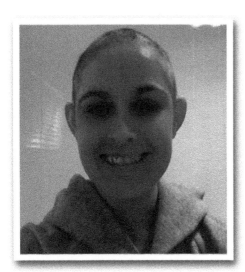

29 July 2012
Lisa at home on the Central Coast, NSW.
She accepted her hair loss
and shaved it off.
"Best decision ever!" – Lisa

Within a few days of treatment, you are also classed as 'immunocompromised'. Your white blood cells drop to buggery, leaving you open to any infection, cold or sniffle going. If you get a temp above 38 Celsius, they admit you to hospital and put you on intravenous antibiotics and fluids as a simple cold can kill you. You may develop neutropenia, meaning you have absolutely no protection from any sickness or illness. That is why you sometimes see cancer patients wearing masks to try to protect themselves from a simple illness that could kill them.

Chemo brain.

When on treatment and afterwards, you can suffer from chemo brain also called chemo fog or chemotherapy-related cognitive impairment. The 'experts' say there is no proof, but until those 'experts' have actually had chemo themselves, I refute their no-evidence finding. Words no longer pop into my head like they used to. I have to sit and think about it for a minute first. I couldn't tell you the amount of times in a day that I ask, "What's that word?" I constantly feel like I have this thick cloud over my head. Crosswords and quiz shows scare me now. Just doing these blogs takes me hours. Before it would have taken me half an hour to write, edit and post, now it's a full-on effort, taking sometimes up to ten hours over a few days. You'll forget simple, everyday things, like you'll ask someone to pass you the salt, but you can't remember the word 'salt'. So you end up just pointing at it and pretending to put salt on your meal until someone understands your charade and they pass you the salt.

Menopause!!!!!

Let the hot flushes and night sweats begin. As previously mentioned, I have now been menopausal three times. Menopause is not fun. Hot flushes come on at any time where a sea of sweat bursts from every pore in your body. One second, you're a perfectly respectable-looking human being, and the next second you look like you've been dunked in a bucket of stinky, sticky sweat with a bright red face to match – not even a nice, gentle glow. You're a bloody beetroot!

The night sweats add to the fact that you're already probably not sleeping well because of the steroids they pump into you when you're on active treatment. You'll be lying in bed in the middle of winter and the next thing it's boiling hot and you're drenched from head to toe. I can't count the amount of times I've had to get out of bed and change my sheets and pyjamas because of night sweats.

Stop reading for the next paragraph, Mum, Dad and any family member!

Sex drive.

Sorry what's that again? I obviously can't speak for everybody, but for me it's non-existent. I'm at a point in a woman's life where sex is apparently at its best, yet I would rather be sitting crocheting with a cup of hot chocolate than have to take my pants off. (I told you I'd write the warts-and-all-story.) I'm including this because it's important. If you're currently going through treatment, in a relationship and probably feeling guilty because you're toxic and certain things are already ruled out for safety reasons – and throw on top of that hormones going berserk – the last thing you want to do is put some Barry White on the iPhone and get some bow-chicka-wow-wow action going. So please don't feel guilty. If your partner doesn't quite get it, explain it to them. If they still don't get it, tell them to read this blog. And if they still don't get it, well, you're stuffed.

You would think that the more chemo you have the easier it gets. In fact, it's the opposite. The more chemo you have, the more it builds up in your system and the sicker you get. Then you get the chemo-anxiety-nausea where you begin to feel sick before you even start the chemo. This is common for chemo patients. Throw in the fact that if you don't have a port (a small catheter under your skin in the chest connected to a vein), your veins begin to collapse. So cannulating for treatment becomes near impossible. It could take four or five attempts to finally get one in. So then you also get cannula anxiety. Oh the joys.

I've had four different types of chemo in my time. They've caused everything from blood clots (so I would have daily heparin injections in my leg or stomach) to burning in the veins, which caused burns on my skin from inside out. My hands and wrists were especially burnt and painful during that treatment, and I had nerve pain in my hands. I couldn't really grip onto anything without pain. For the burning and rashes, I found MooGoo creams brilliant. They have a huge range and are available in most chemists. Or you can purchase them online directly from moogoo.com.au.(No, I'm not being paid for the endorsement!)

I'm sorry to any of you out there that perhaps googled chemo side effects and happened across my blog, looking for some positives. It's a shit show from beginning to end, and once you've actually completed treatment, people don't understand it takes months to years for the body to reboot. It's just been through the biggest war ever, and a bit of PTSD should be expected not to mention the long-term effects that many are left with for life. Some people suffer from nerve damage and are in constant discomfort once completing treatment. Then there's infertility, osteoporosis, liver problems, lung disease, and the list goes on.

So to sum it all up, chemo is SHITTY.

The end!

Peter and I were in Queensland many times when Lisa was having chemo after her first diagnosis. We thought that staying with Lisa and her partner would add further stress to an already difficult situation. It really was a balancing act. How could we spend time with Lisa and help her get through the toughest days without making life more difficult for her? We treasured the last two years of life with Lisa. But we live with a lot of regret for all the times we couldn't be there. You can speak to someone on the telephone ten times a day, but it is not the same as sitting, holding their hand.

I will never understand how anyone goes through cancer alone. As much as they may say they don't need help or support, they truly do, even if it is just hand holding. As a carer of *Don't ask, just do.* someone with a terminal illness, if I can give friends and family one piece of advice it would be this: Don't ask, just do. Take over a casserole, make a cup of tea, or do a little ironing or house cleaning. Most people will never tell you what they need. They don't like to put others out. I remember the simple pleasure of having a cup of tea made for me. It was absolutely the best feeling ever getting something handed to me. It made me take time for a chat and took away the feeling of isolation and loneliness. I treasured it.

My advice to anyone that has a loved one going through the cancer journey is to stay close. Forget silly little arguments and ignore the trivial things that would generally annoy you. Just be there for your loved one.

Friendships Forge Survival: My Friends' Perspective

01/04/2016

Friend: *a person with whom one has a bond of mutual affection, typically one exclusive of sexual or family relations.*

Friendship: *the emotions or conduct of friends; the state of being friends.*

Friends play a huge role in any person's life, but especially in women's lives. They are our confidants, our sounding boards, and almost like our priests who you can swear at, if you will.

Friends provide us with the type of love and support that a family member or even a partner can't. A lot of that I feel has to do with honesty, and that honesty doesn't always come without judgement. In fact, much of the time a friendship holds a lot of judgement; well, my friendships do. I prefer my friend to tell me that I'm being an idiot, or that I do look fat in that dress. I want my friend to trust in our relationship enough that she/he feels safe and confident enough to say whatever they want without me 'unfriending' them, so to speak.

I'm not saying that there haven't been times where a friend has said or done something that has upset or even angered me. Of course, we've had our spats; that's healthy in any relationship. If you haven't had some sort of disagreement in a long-term friendship, I suggest you haven't always been completely honest with your friend about your feelings. For me life is too short to bullshit to someone just to make them feel better. In saying that, the odd occasion where you've told me that that blinder of a pimple that's been guiding flight VA815 into Brisbane airport for the last couple of nights isn't that noticeable is acceptable friendship fudging. It's a delicate dance this friendship business.

I would say that most people say they choose their friends because of who 'they' are, and they select them because they have common interests. You might both do yoga and talking to each other is easy. Or maybe you both like to down a bottle of wine every night. Whatever that commonality may be, that is why you're friends. But I believe we remain friends with people for extended periods because of the way they support who 'we' are. We remain friends because they love 'us' for our warts and all. How ᴄ supports 'us', I believe, plays a huge part in the longevity of a friena. not the little things like a joint love of BoxSets and Botox. It's because th, friendship makes us feel good about ourselves.

I went through a long period, due to personal reasons, where I didn't communicate with my friends as often as I should have. Because of that I lost many. But there were the ones who stuck (when I certainly wouldn't have), and for that I am grateful. They are the ones who still stick by me through thick and thin. They've been with me through break-ups, work problems, cancer, chemo, treatments and weight gain/weight loss. Even when I wasn't as active a friend as I should be, they persisted. Now that I've realised how important friendships are, and even though I live in a whole different state to them, we see each other more often than we did when I lived around the corner from them.

Each of my friends are from completely different backgrounds and very different personalities. But the funny thing is, on the very odd occasions that we've all gotten together, we all meld. It's amazing. They all have one thing in common – me and their genuine love for me – which I say makes me a pretty lucky person.

So what's this blog about? I asked a small handful of my best friends to answer these questions:

- How did you feel when you found out I was terminal?
- How do you cope?
- Has it affected our relationship?

So here are some of their responses, in their words.

Nicole:

When I first heard Lisa had cancer, it didn't seem as though I heard or processed it, more like I felt it. Like you feel a punch in the sternum. It feels more like an ache now. The surprise from the punch is gone, but it feels the same.

I feel the same way about Lisa now as I did prior to diagnosis, for the most part. I don't think Lisa would want it any other way. I think one of the things we both enjoy about our friendship is the unfiltered honesty.

I think the only differences are that I find myself in awe of her strength of character and attitude towards this fight. Lisa has remarkable spirit and maintains a filthy sense of humour. Her ability to keep positive in the face of cancer has made me look at my trials from a different perspective. I'm very thankful for that.

> Lisa has remarkable spirit and maintains a filthy sense of humour.

A terminal diagnosis is obviously devastating, and I deal with it by doing what I think is my 'job': to just keep being the same friend. It is not about me and how I feel. Lisa has enough on her plate without worrying about how I am dealing with what is her own, very personal position. You can't just take the good stuff. I'm trying to balance being positive with allowing Lisa to speak openly to me about how she is feeling when she is struggling with treatment, scared or overwhelmed. It's a privilege to be a confidant.

Of course, I think it's a shit hand and incredibly unfair. I get angry about it and find myself devastated when I hear a treatment hasn't been effective or tumours have grown. I try not to dwell on the diagnosis when I think about Lisa though. It does not define who she is to me.

Rebecca:

We all have that one friend you share your everything with — that one friend who is the missing piece to your puzzle. So what would happen if you lost them? If they were no longer at the other end of the phone like you were used to? This is the question that plays through my mind day in and day out.

That moment when Lisa rang to deliver the news that her cancer was back was like being thrown under a bus. Seriously, give a girl a break. This can't be happening. Instantly my reaction was "Let's just fix it", but the reality is it's not just a broken heart, a wrongly purchased dress or the realisation that either one of us had gained a kilo. It is cancer: We can't fix this!!!!

TERMINALLY *fabulous*

How do you stay brave for someone when you are barely coping with the idea yourself? Sometimes I feel like it is Lisa who is holding it together for all of us, which in turn keeps us strong. The only thing I could promise was that I would refuse to let cancer define our friendship. We have been friends for close on 20 years, and while everything is changing around her, I don't want our friendship to be one of them. For that reason, I do my best not to talk chemo, tumour size and death, but I instead continue to talk nail polish, fashion, boys, love and all those other things only best friends have the answer to. Don't get me wrong. We also talk fear, anger, funerals and bucket lists. But every moment I can, I go back to the normal stuff. I guess it's my way of keeping my best friend as my best friend for as long as I can, rather than losing her to cancer before I have to.

Then there is the other side of this. I refuse to accept that one day, way before we had planned, I am not going to have my best friend around. To be honest the thought scares the shit out of me!!!

She believed she could, so she did!!!

Our saying is, "She believed she could, so she did!!!" I love her!!! Xxx

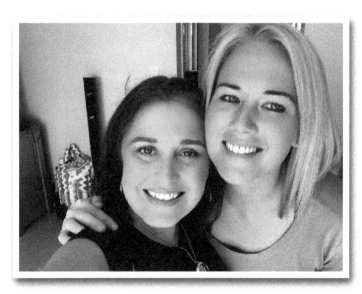

23 May 2016
A wee visit from Lisa's bestie Rebecca Cooper... just what the doctor ordered.

Melissa:

When you were diagnosed, I had no doubt in my mind that you would be cured. A bit of surgery and chemo and you'd be all good. Selfishly, I didn't think that someone else I loved could possibly die from this arsehole of a disease, when so many people fight it and survive. I can't remember my reaction when you told me it was terminal. But I would assume the word 'fuck' was involved.

I always wanted to be someone you could be honest with about how you were feeling. I hope I have been that.

How do I cope? In all honesty I am not sure I do at times. Many a tear has been shed for you when I am sitting alone at home with time to think. I cope by talking to you and having a laugh. I cope by talking to Mum and having a cry. I scream at the world and ask that question we all have — WHY?? But at the end of the day, it is you who are suffering. If I can play any small part in making your life better, however long it may be, I will do whatever I can.

Love you xx

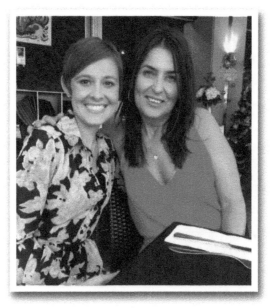

A beautiful visit from a very close friend Kieran Macri.
2nd January 2015 at Hope Island QLD.

TERMINALLY *fabulous*

Sharon:

Hearing that your cancer had returned and was terminal left me feeling immediate denial and confusion. I cried, and I was pissed off. How dare that cancer rear its ugly head again!!

I know it sounds cliché, but I seriously changed my entire outlook and attitude. You inspired me to get off my arse and change my journey to appreciate the 'little' things. So many times a day I motivate myself to stop thinking, stop procrastinating, stop questioning. I have a no-nonsense approach to my life now.

How do I feel about you? I feel blessed and thankful that our paths crossed. You are a force to be reckoned with, and I'm pissed off that cancer chose to mess with you. I feel that your guts and determination are your greatest attributes. You, my friend, have taught me so much about myself. Before you came into my life, I did have this battered little person inside continually second guessing herself and looking for recognition and praise. You are my inspiration. Yes, cliché but it's true. I adore you xx

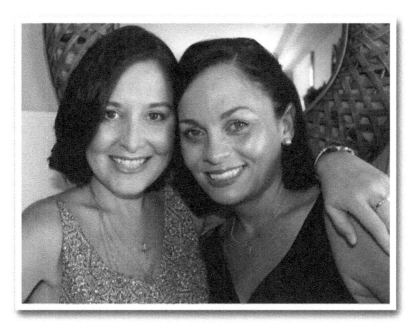

15 February 2016
Lisa and Sharon Glasson during a girls' weekend
away at Broadbeach, Gold Coast, QLD.

So there you have it: a small insight into how friends are affected by this disease.

For those friends out there who are trying to figure out the best way to deal with a friend having cancer, the best advice I can give is to take off the kid gloves. We are still the same person we were yesterday. Don't constantly be repeating clichés like 'We'll beat this' or 'It'll all be fine'. Yes, of course we want to hear that we can get through this – unless we're terminal. Then the old 'They're coming up with new things everyday' bullshit really gets on my goat.

But we also want you to express your fear, your sadness. I sometimes have felt alienated or somewhat of a hypochondriac. When I'm bald and have no eyelashes and eyebrows and you still insist on telling me you don't notice and I'm still beautiful, it infuriates me. I want you to say the truth. I want you to say, "Yes, you do resemble Dan Aykroyd from his *Coneheads* days without eyebrows". And when I'm on the floor in a ball crying from pain or chemo side effects, I don't want you to just hug me and say it'll all be alright. If you want to cry, please cry. Sometimes we just need you to lie on the floor next to us and cry and break down too. In some strange way, it makes us feel better.

For those who want to help but don't want to be the emotionally-supportive one, offer to bring over cooked food, pick up prescriptions for them, do a bit of laundry, clean their house, offer to babysit or pick up the kids after school. These things will help greatly and be beneficial to both you and your friend.

Some friends will distance themselves from you because they simply cannot deal with it. If you're one of those people, text your friend and tell them why you've gone AWOL. We will most likely understand, but don't just disappear.

As I've said before, this disease does not just affect the patient. So for you, the one with cancer, try to be gentle on your friend. They're trying to navigate this minefield as well. It's new territory for everyone. So lower your friendship expectations for a little while, until your friend has time to digest everything and come to terms (if that's ever possible) with the fact that you could be facing death.

Most of all, like with any friendship, honesty is the best policy. Speak with your friend when things have settled down a bit about how you want your friendship to work during this arsehole of a journey, sort of like a game plan – a friendship plan. That way you both know where you're at and where you're coming from. It may sound silly, but I feel facing it head-on early on, and making each other aware of both your expectations, will help you avoid a lot of stress and heartache down the road. There is no right or wrong way to handle it. You're both going to be scared and unsure of what the future may hold. So be gentle on each other.

All I've ever wanted from my friends, pre-cancer and now, is support and unconditional love. And that's what they've given me. I am truly lucky that I have each of my friends to ring and cry to when I feel like shit and can't face the next day. Or when I want to bitch or to talk about last night's episode of *Beverly Hills Housewives*. So basically, a friendship before cancer is exactly the same as during cancer and terminal cancer. It's just that it probably holds a bit more meaning than it did before.

> A friendship before cancer is exactly the same as during cancer and terminal cancer.

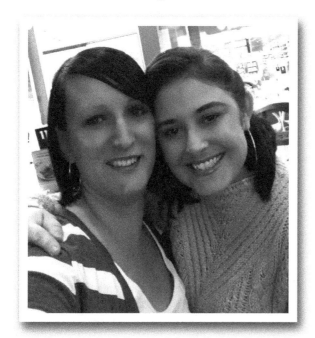

18 June 2016
Lisa and Mel Grand
at Coffee Club,
Springfield Central,
during a treasured
fly-in visit by Mel.

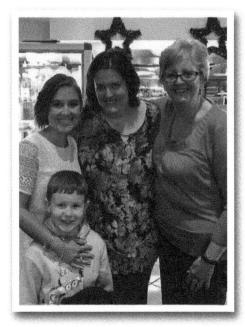

A lovely catch up with friends who have become family. Mel Holly, her beautiful boy Alex and her dear mum Margaret Buffrey. 15th November 2015, Penrith NSW.

Thank you to my friends who provided their responses. And thank you to those other friends of mine who are there for me no matter what. Your love and support are a large part of what has seen me through the days where I just don't think I can fight anymore. You guys are the ones who make me get back in the ring again.

One thing Peter and I will be eternally grateful for is Lisa's circle of friends. Not only did they support Lisa, but they also supported our family, me in particular. They still do. Because Lisa was so open with them, she would tell them everything that was going on. They knew when she was having a bad day and why. I always knew when Lisa had been talking to them as not long afterwards, I would receive a message from them asking how I was. They would always reassure me that I was doing the right thing and give me the encouragement I needed to get back on the horse. They believed in me when I didn't believe in myself.

Many times during Lisa's illness, the girls would get that nightmare phone call when we thought Lisa wouldn't make it through the night. There was never doubt nor hesitation; they were always on the next flight. The girls never once complained about flying up to see Lisa. But I would often hesitate before I called them. As frantic and worried as I was, I became a little complacent. I would have the little voice at the back of my mind reminding me that we'd been here before, and Lisa would surely once again show cancer who it was dealing with and turn a corner. But in the end, I would make the dreaded calls and one by one the girls would arrive.

My friendship with the girls strengthened with each visit. Other than our family and a couple of very close friends, they were the only ones I could leave Lisa with to have a break whilst they were visiting. So they became a bit of a lifeline for me.

They care for us even though they are hurting too. Rebecca, Lisa's best friend, struggles daily. Like us, all she wants is Lisa back. Sharon feels so isolated as she lives at the other side of Australia, but she never lets a week

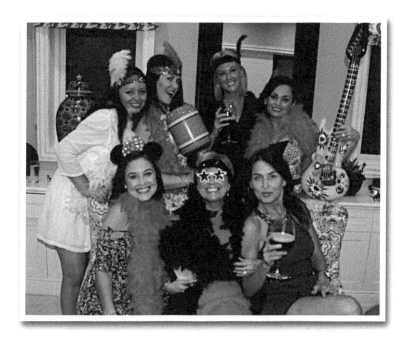

13 February 2016
Dress-up fun on a girls' weekend away at Broadbeach, Gold Coast.
Back row: Aleana McGuiness, Marianne, Rebecca Cooper, Sharon Glasson.
Front row: Lisa, Geraldine, Kieran Macri.

go by without contact. Nicole is the silent rock of support. She has done so many kind things for me out of the blue and without grand public announcements. She reminds me of Lisa in many ways. Kieran, Mel (by two) and so many more are our guardian angels in disguise.

Now that Lisa has passed nothing has changed; they call, they message, and they visit. I know I can turn to any of them on the toughest of days and they will always listen.

I remember our family from Ireland worrying because we were going through this nightmare without them being close enough to support us. I would always reassure them that we had a great support network here. Pete and I don't have a massive friendship circle, but the friends we do have are like Lisa's friends: one call and they'll be here.

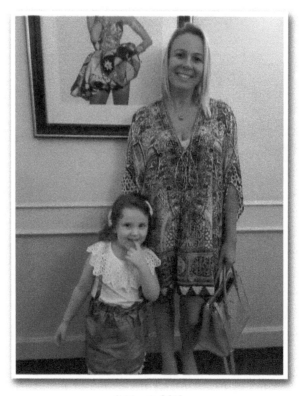

11 March 2018
Nicole Onesti and Ava at the Palazzo Versace, Gold
Coast, on the first anniversary of Lisa's passing

The New Normal: Living While You Are Dying

05/04/2016

I had to enter a calendar entry for a chest CAT scan for tomorrow morning and noticed a previous calendar entry on the 6th of April 2012. It was the date I was initially told I had a massive tumour on my stomach. That was my first foray into hearing the C-word in 'my' world. The reminder came up at the perfect time as I was thinking, *What in the hell am I going to blog about next?* Then the calendar heaven gates opened and gave me my 'cancerversary' as I like to call it.

So this blog is about 'living' while you're 'dying'. Yes, I know, and I've heard it all before: "We're all dying. I could walk off the gutter tomorrow and be hit by a bus." Um sorry? When was the last time you put on the news and saw that someone was hit by a bus? Maybe I'm just more sensitive to it because of my situation, but I can only speak for myself. And my truth is that prior to cancer and a terminal cancer diagnosis, I was always thinking or saying, "That's okay. I can do it tomorrow" or "We can go on that once in a lifetime holiday next year" or "I can see my best friend at Christmas, which is four months away".

Because we don't think about our mortality daily, I was always putting things off. But if you don't know if you'll be here next week, next month or next year, you start to think differently about living. It's like having the grim reaper constantly peering over your shoulder.

Some people hear the word 'terminal' and immediately start dying. They give up. True to the oncologist's prognosis, they won't make three months. I'm not saying that if they had tried chemo or started chanting to Buddha, or started thinking positive affirmations or meditating, that they would have lasted six months. I am obviously no higher power, so I don't hold the key to what makes one person with the same cancer and prognosis live two months and another nine years. I have no idea; nobody does. It is an individual thing.

When faced with a person in the oncology waiting room who recently received a terminal prognosis, this is why I always say, "Don't listen to the doctor. They don't know. They're just giving you answers based on statistics not on your determination to fight".

I'm also not saying that just because you say, "I'm going to beat these odds. I'm going to prove this bastard cancer wrong", and you wake up every morning positive about your outcome, that you will extend your time on earth. Or that you can achieve every terminal cancer patient's dream of the elusive miracle cure. I can only go on what I think has helped 'me'. Positivity, hope and prayer (mixed with a few toxic potions and radiation now and then) have greatly helped me.

> Positivity, hope and prayer have greatly helped me.

STRESS! I truly believe stress plays a huuuuuge part in EVERY person's health, not just a terminally-ill person's life. For a terminal person stress management is imperative. You have to face your prognosis head-on and not put your head in the sand. You have to let it scare you before you can find coping mechanisms to deal with it. Then you hopefully accept it and learn to 'live' with it rather than 'die prematurely' from it.

Some people find counselling hugely beneficial. I didn't. I've been to a few counsellors over the years and felt like I could help myself more than they could help me. That's not to say it won't work for you. So I always suggest trying it first, even trying a few different counsellors. You may find one that works for you, which is great. Only yesterday I started to speak with a chaplain that my community nurse recommended, and for the first time in a 'session' I got it. She was great, and I plan on seeing her again. It's just an added bonus that she actually comes to your house, so you don't even need to apply concealer.

Another tip that you think would be universally known but isn't: Don't wear mascara to your counselling session!

If there are people or situations in your life that cause you anxiety on top of your already stressful situation, you need to address it. Maybe let your friend know that her constantly crying and mourning you before you're dead doesn't help your stress levels. Stresses that existed before your prognosis also don't just disappear. Your credit card debt, your unhealthy relationship and your argument with your mum about where you're spending Christmas don't just disappear into thin air. You still have to deal with the same everyday stresses as everybody else. So I definitely advise addressing these issues before they make you sicker

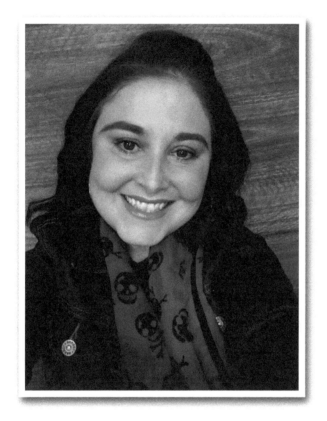

29 June 2016
Lisa at Mater Hospital, Springfield Lakes, QLD, before her lung CAT scan.

Another important aspect of a terminal diagnosis is getting your affairs in order. It's something no-one really ever wants to do. Who wants to organise their own funeral? But it is what it is, especially if you don't want to leave that added stress for your loved ones. I recommend at least defining your wishes clearly in your will and testament. Again, I know you don't want to as it feels a bit like you're giving in. But honestly, it's not that. It's being organised. It's actually recommended that once you get married, have children or buy a house you should organise a will. So if you haven't already, get on it!

When organising your will, you can also organise your will executor (the person who looks after a person's wishes once they die) and your attorney (this person has power of attorney to manage your affairs, including financial, while you are alive). Your will and power of attorney are both legally binding documents that remove the stress from your loved ones as decisions have already been made.

Another thing a terminal patient should organise for both themselves and their carers or family is an advance healthcare directive. It's basically a living will that stipulates what should happen to you, healthwise, if you can no longer communicate your choice or if you're no longer able to make decisions for yourself (like should you be resuscitated or ventilated). It's a great thing to have signed copies that are authenticated by a JP for your GP: one for your carer or attorney, one for when and if an ambulance comes to your house and a few extras that you can hand out at the hospital if need be.

People often say they admire me or I inspire them to live differently. That's great. It's nice to know that some good can come from such an absolutely shitty situation. They often say, "I don't know how you do it. How do you still find the good in life? How are you still able to smile and laugh?"

My response is simply "You don't know what you're made of until you're faced with it".

If you had asked me prior to prognosis how I'd handle hearing that I'm dying much sooner than I should be, I'd have said that I would probably crawl into a ball and die. But I haven't. Instead I have stood tall. I've faced my fears head-on. I've made some changes to my life. One of the best things I ever did was relocating up north to be close to my family. They play such a huge part in my life, and they want to support me through this. All in all, I've surprised myself at how I've dealt with it. I say yes to lunch with that long-lost friend now, instead of saying we'll catch up next time. I now buy tickets to shows that aren't on for three months now and don't give it a second thought. I'm either here for it or I'm not.

One thing I want to make clear before I sign off is that I'm not always stoic. I'm not always this strong, positive person. I have my moments, where a treatment has not worked or my pain levels are high, when I do cry and say I'm scared.

When you're first given the prognosis you may look at people with jealousy. Why is that woman a healthy mum? Why is that old lady 85 and never been in hospital? Why me? Why have I been burdened with this?

You might often think about things in timelines like:

- I'm not going to be here next Christmas.
- Could this be the last time I see my aunty?
- I'm not going to be here to see my niece start school.

These thoughts have dwindled over the years for me. I don't think about them every day like I did initially. Now they're just random thoughts, which is good. It means I'm living, not prematurely dying.

> It means I'm living, not prematurely dying.

Helping Lisa organise her funeral and will were extremely difficult for me. But I had no other option. Lisa was hurting as it was, and not having it taken care of was stressing her out. I knew I had to park my personal feelings and get on with it. One piece of advice I would give anyone is do it sooner rather than later. Don't wait for a terminal diagnosis. In fact, don't wait until you have a serious illness; just do it.

When Lisa was originally diagnosed and was having surgery to remove the tumour, I promised myself that when she was back on her feet and fighting fit, I would sit down with both her and Steven and ask them what their wishes were should anything ever happen to them. Peter and I would also tell them what we each wanted should anything happen to us. When Lisa was between treatments and her pain was being well-controlled, I suggested we get the advance health directive and will out of the way. Even if we never had to use it, it would be done.

The reality was Peter and I both knew it would be needed, but if I had said it with urgency Lisa would have become stressed. I wasn't worried about the will, but I was worried about the health directive. Prior to it being completed, I would worry that when Lisa was rushed to hospital, if she didn't make it we had no idea what she wanted. Or if she was unconscious, we wouldn't know what decision to make on her health if needed.

Thankfully, the social worker from palliative care helped with this process. She explained the stages of disease progression and the impact of resuscitation at each stage. For example, if the cancer had spread throughout the body and CPR was used, the repercussions on the patient could be drastic. These were the types of things we needed to discuss.

If you take one piece of advice from this book, please let this be it: Get that paperwork sorted.

Remember, these discussions and documents are even more important when partners are involved. It's not about the partner and it's not about the parent; it's about the patient. It's also important to keep the documentation updated should something change that would impact your health directive, for example, disease progression. This is what your medical team will work off should you be unconscious and unable to speak for yourself. It's always better to make such decisions when your head is clear, your pain levels under control and you have the time to consider what your wishes would be under different circumstances.

The Big What If

09/04/2016

What if?

It's a question that I've often found myself asking. I try not to because if you keep looking back, you can't move forward.

My story: Upon my initial diagnosis I was directed by my GP to go to a particular surgeon. So being the obedient patient that I am, and because doctors are 'God', I toddled off to the surgeon she suggested.

This surgeon suggested I had a GIST – a gastrointestinal stromal tumour. This is a 'good' one to get as it's a sarcoma that the medical field know about. It also has a treatment drug called Imatinib in tablet form, a tyrosine-kinase inhibitor that is good to take after having your tumour removed. It blocks the enzyme that allows cancer to grow – an added security blanket to help prevent the cancer from returning.

After quite a wait – three months! – pathologists determined that my cancer had a similar appearance to sarcoma. So they decided to call it an undifferentiated gastric sarcoma. Sarcoma accounts for less than one per cent of cancers diagnosed each year, so it's rare already. So mine is incredibly rare. In fact, one of a kind. Unique, just like me. Any surgeon who has performed a sarcoma tumour removal should know that you need to take more out than less. Be aggressive and remove more, or all, of the stomach. Just take that arsehole out and make sure you take its little cancerous mates with it.

My original surgeon was a laparoscopic surgeon with no experience with sarcoma resection. But I didn't know that at the time. He directed me to an oncologist at the same hospital, and once again I followed his advice blindly. I didn't question anything. I just did what I was told. Upon completion of chemotherapy, my oncologist recommended further surgery. They call this a 'whoops' surgery as he said I didn't have 'clear' margins after my initial surgery. Once again, I returned to the first surgeon and had more of my stomach removed. This time the pathology came back as cancer free.

My reason for revisiting all of this is to help educate you on what you should do when you first find out you have cancer. If you are told what type of cancer you have (from biopsy results, blood tests etc), investigate different specialists who specialise in that particular type of cancer. When my cancer came back, I visited three different oncologists and a couple of surgeons.

When you meet with them question, question, question!!!!! First, ask if you can record the conversation. When you are speaking with the oncologist, you are already in a daze, so you most likely are not going to be listening properly. They will use big words and words

When you meet with them question, question, question!!!!!

that you've never heard before. So recording the conversation allows you to sit back and review it and absorb it. Take a list of questions into the consultation with you because you will forget most of them. Your emotions are high and you're still in shock. So it's great to have them written down and tick them off as you go.

What type of questions should you ask? Here's a handy list:

- What kind of cancer do I have?
- Do you specialise in my type of cancer?
- Can I be cured?
- What stage is it?
- Is it localised, or has it spread?
- Is it a common cancer?
- What treatments, if any, do I need to have?
- Will the treatments improve my chance of survival?
- Are there different treatment options; if so, what are the pros and cons of each?
- Where will I have treatment?
- What are the side effects of treatment?
- How long will I require treatment for?
- Are there any clinical trials; if so, would it be worth it for me to try one?
- Are there any things you recommend getting done before treatment, like freezing my eggs or having a needle that helps prevent menopause during chemo? *(something I wasn't made aware of)*
- Are there long-term side effects?
- Are there any costs involved?
- Do you have any literature or statistics about my cancer?
- Is there someone I can talk to such as a counsellor or even a person who has previously had this treatment or cancer?
- What is the best-case scenario and the worst-case scenario?

These are just a few questions that you should ask of potential oncologists. These questions can also be asked if you need to speak with a radiation oncologist. Most importantly, DO NOT feel railroaded into choosing a certain oncologist. Just because your doctor likes them doesn't mean they're the best fit for you. Remember, you're going to be having a very personal relationship with this person. So apart from the fact that you want them to know what they're doing, you also want to feel comfortable talking to each other. You should be able to tell your oncologist ANYTHING!

This is not like buying a dress. You can't return bad or incorrect treatment. This is your life and this person literally holds it in their hands. So it's imperative that you feel safe and comfortable with them. I cannot stress enough that it's not like choosing a hairdresser, although I know on the scale of importance a good hairdresser rates very highly, as too does a good eyebrow waxer. But unlike hair, your survival will not grow back. You need to make sure you come ready to fight, and to do this, you have to have a fantastic support team, a medical entourage if you will.

Information is also one of the best weapons you can take into your cancer fight. So ask for up-to-date information from the Cancer Council, your oncologist and your cancer centre. Google safely and sensibly. Some people like to know nothing and just leave it all in the specialists' hands. That approach doesn't work for me. I need to know all there is to know. But at the end of the day, whether you want to know or not, it's your decision. We all handle things differently. Don't let anybody tell you how you should handle this. This is your story; tell it the way you want.

Depending on your cancer you may also require a surgeon. As I mentioned earlier, it is hugely important that you ask the right questions to get the best surgeon for your case. Although many cancers have the same or similar pathology, every case is still individual. You want your surgeon to treat you as that – an individual.

Most of the questions above can be applied to surgery, but you need to ask things like:

- Do you specialise in this type of cancer surgery?
- How many of these surgeries have you performed successfully and otherwise?
- Have you seen my specific type of cancer and positioning before?
- What type of surgery will you be performing?
- How long will you be in surgery?
- What are the risks of the surgery?

- Will there be any long-term effects after surgery, such as will I need a colostomy bag, or will I lose a limb or an organ?
- Do I have to have surgery?
- Will you be performing the surgery; if not who will be? *(Quite often people visit a surgeon and then, when they're operated on, one of the registrars performs the surgery. So if you want them to specifically do it, make sure you confirm that they're performing it.)*
- What effects should I expect after surgery?
- How long will I be in hospital?
- How long will my recovery take?

I don't want you to be in the position I was in where I just rushed into everything and didn't investigate anything. Doctors will tell you NOT to google. I agree that you can be misled by googling, but it can also be an effective tool in your cancer treatment. You can google specialists, surgeons, trials, cancer descriptions and much more. But be aware that when you google 'cancer', you're going to get some hairy results. So if you're not prepared to see things you don't want to see, DON'T DO IT!!!!!

This is your body. More than that, this is your LIFE. Cancer is not a game. I know that when you're first diagnosed, everything feels urgent. Sometimes it is. My cancer needed to be treated ASAP, but I still could have looked into different specialists and treatment options. Give yourself a couple of days to let it start to sink in, and then investigate different specialists and treatment centres. Maybe speak to someone you know who's had cancer and get their advice. Look at chatrooms in relation to your cancer. Cancer Council Australia is a great place to start. They have so much advice and also have a Find a Specialist section www.cancer.org.au/about-cancer/find-a-specialist.html.

> Get the best team members you can get to win the most important game of your life.

'You have cancer' are three of the scariest words you could ever hear. So allow yourself to freak out. Allow yourself to scream, cry and hate the world. But then you need to put your big girl/boy pants on and face this beast head-on. Get the best team members you can get to win the most important game of your life. You must feel confident that the

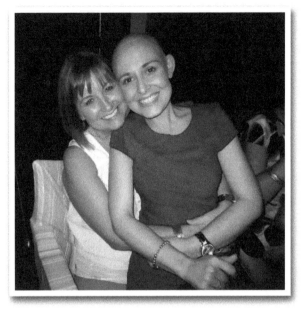

25 January 2014
Lisa and her mum, Geraldine Magill, at Forster, NSW, celebrating Lisa's 32nd birthday, two weeks before major surgery and still on chemotherapy.

people in your team are the best for you and that they all have one end game – your survival.

Don't end up like me, asking "What if?"

What Happens When 3 Months Drag On and On

14/04/2016

When you've had a cancer diagnosis, it stays with you, probably forever. Life toddles on, but it's never the same again. I can't speak for others, but maybe as time goes on cancer disappears from one's thoughts. I've heard that with each clear scan it becomes easier, but the cancer cloud still manages to hover over your head now and then and rain on your parade. It doesn't storm on you every day, though, like it does early on after completing treatment.

As I only had nine months of NED (No Evidence of Disease), I know that it was still very raw. In fact, in December 2012 (less than a month after my final treatment), my brother Steven and his wife Marianne announced their pregnancy. I did my best to act happy and excited for them, but inside I was a mess. My first thought was *That's it, I'm going to die. The old one-in-one-out thing. He/she will be my replacement. My cancer is going to come back. I'm going to die!*

I eventually divulged to Steven what my whole reaction was about, and he understood, which was good for me. I then dove into organising baby showers, craft for the nursery and so on.

As the story goes, a week after Ava's birth, I got the news that my cancer was back. And this time around it was incurable. I went to four different oncologists, as I wasn't happy with my initial treatment, and shopped around. I was told by each of them, bar one, that I would be lucky to make it to three months. I was offered numerous scary procedures and chemotherapies to extend my life by maybe months, not years.

I knew the oncologist that I eventually chose from one of my BFF's sisters who had recently passed away from recurring Ewing's sarcoma. He told her straight up that there was nothing they could do for her and to basically go home and die. So when I met him, and he told me there was hope and the possibility of cure was there, I knew he wouldn't under-exaggerate or over-exaggerate my chances at a longer survival. I picked him to be my treating oncologist. I know that without him and his positivity and treatments I would not still be here two-and-a-half years later.

Under him, I was given three different chemos, a couple of immunotherapies, a massive debulking surgery that other hospitals and surgeons refused to do and eight radiation therapies. Here I am, still holding on by the edge of my fingernails, but I'm here. I partly put that down to his positive attitude, which in turn lifted my spirits and made me positive. Prior to that all I could think was *I'm dying. I'm not going to be here next Christmas. I'm not going to get to see the next series of* Homeland. *I'm not going to see Ava grow up. I'm never going to get married or have kids* and so on.

I'm now at that point where we've run out of options other than radiation. And we won't see results of my recent radiation treatment for another four weeks. But the funny thing is that because I'm still here, I sometimes think that people are thinking or saying, "What is going on with her? Wasn't she meant to be dead like years ago? Is she really as sick as she says she is? Is she even dying?"

I really think people must be confused. I also get worried that they see that I'm complaining about pain or being in a wheelchair from time to time, and then they see me at the tennis and think *Hang on a minute. She was in hospital two days ago and now she's in Melbourne at the tennis. It doesn't make sense.* The fact of the matter is I am in pain 24/7. It's just that sometimes the pain is completely unmanageable, and I have to go to hospital or sit in the wheelchair to conserve my energy.

I spend most days in pain but pretending that I'm not, for other people's sakes. I have weekly palliative nurse and community nurse visits. I take numerous meds morning and night and inject pain relief up to five or six times a day. I visit oncologists' offices and get treatments in cold, sterile cancer wards (although the staff and nurses in most of these places are warm, caring and inviting). People imagine you start a bucket list and go over to Disneyland or on safari in Africa. You get to meet Beyoncé backstage at her concert or fly over to New York and spend Christmas there, or you skydive. It's just not like that.

Firstly, where does the money come from? The reality is, if you have terminal cancer you can't get insurance. So going overseas is an expensive exercise. If you get ill over there, it's at your own expense. Sometimes your oncologist refuses to support you going overseas. For me the risk of bleeding out on the flight, or not getting the best treatment available if I go to some exotic island, is too risky for my oncologist to support. So going to NYC at Christmas time is not doable. I actually had tickets to Vegas booked and front-table VIP Britney Spears tickets, but I had to cancel my trip just days out because of anal bleeding. If you have tumours like me, you can't safely go skydiving or tightrope walking or even bowling! Seriously, I'm not allowed to roll a ball down a lane at pins because of the weight of the ball! I can't go on the rides at Disneyland even if I was allowed to fly to LA. So the idea of a bucket list is great, but it's just not always doable.

People think you get sympathy freebies if you mention the C-word. "Did you mention you have terminal cancer, so you can get upgraded to a suite at the hotel?" It's not like you're a newly-married couple and they upgrade you on your flight or give you the honeymoon suite. If it does work like that, I've been missing out on these cancer benefits. People look at me funny when I park in a disability car parking spot. I don't drive often as I suffer from micro sleeps sometimes, and it's not safe for me to be driving more than 20 minutes at a time. I sometimes use the disability toilet to inject my pain meds as they're more likely to have a sharps container. Quite often, though, sharps containers aren't available, which is ludicrous.

I can't get a job because, let's be honest, if you're applying for a job, they ask you if you have any illnesses that may affect your ability to work. "Um, does terminal cancer count?" So I don't have a job as a creative outlet. I don't get that feeling of achievement from working. I simply fill my days with blogs, doctors' appointments, scans, selfies and babysitting my niece. The fact that my two-and-a-half-year-old niece tells her family child carer that Lisa has a sore belly and is in hospital (even when I'm not) speaks volumes. Poor Ava has spent more time in hospitals than in parks.

I will not allow those people (if any) out there that question my legitimacy get to me. I know my illness. I know the seriousness and daily risks that I face. My life is not all tennis games and handbags. It's more IVs and nurses. On those occasions that I get to go out and enjoy myself, even if I am in my wheelchair, I won't feel guilty for that. I will continue to force myself to go out because people don't understand that I actually have to make myself go out as I have chronic fatigue from radiation and other treatments. I will continue to do things that I enjoy whilst I am still capable of doing so.

> Live every day like you're dying tomorrow.

So yes, I am still terminal, as we all are really. And I intend to still be terminally fabulous for many years to come. My advice to everyone is to live every day like you're dying tomorrow. It will make you appreciate each day more, and maybe make your life count that little bit more.

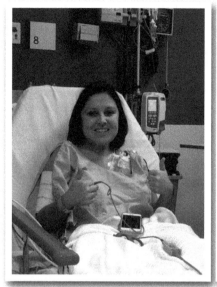 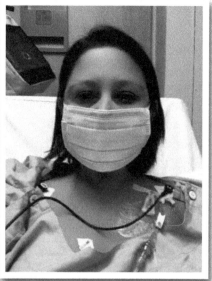

15 April 2016
Another hospital stay for
Lisa at Greenslopes Private
Hospital, Brisbane, QLD.

21 April 2016
The hospital stay continues at
Greenslopes Private Hospital.

Marianne getting pregnant was always going to stir up mixed emotions for Lisa. However, I think Lisa would agree that Ava was sent for a reason. I don't believe Lisa would have survived as long as she did because as Ava continued to grow, Lisa's determination to hit certain milestones really took over. Ava lived the first three-and-a-half years of her life knowing that Lisa was ill. When the time was near, she was told that Lisa would be going to heaven to be an angel. Lisa loved her so much, and they were very close. Losing Lisa was never going to be easy for Ava, no matter how well she was prepared.

One thing is for sure: no-one knew Lisa's body and treatment like Lisa. She knew all the terminology, the full names and abbreviated names of every medication she was on and every after effect, as mentioned above. She would always double check all the information anyone gave her on Google. Quite often she was right to do so as it proved to be beneficial and prepared her for what lay ahead.

Later in her journey, one of the greatest challenges Lisa and I had was her need to control everything. Even when she was so ill and weak, she struggled to let go. Earlier, though, I was so glad that Lisa was the way she was. As she mentioned, cancer was a whole new world that we'd never experienced. Some of the words and terminology were foreign to us but not to Lisa. When we left each appointment, she would explain to me what was said and what it meant. She was always ahead of the game. Even though we initially had no idea of who specialised in what, it didn't take Lisa long to get to grips with sarcoma and become an expert in it. She questioned everything about her medication, treatment plan and both her long- and short-term prognoses. If she didn't feel she got an answer, or she didn't understand the answer, she questioned again.

If it doesn't look right or feel right, it isn't right.

I think we often forget that medical practitioners are human. A doctor can make a slip of the tongue, and a nurse can become comfortable with distributing medication. If it doesn't look right or feel right, it isn't right. Lisa was absolutely on top of her care. I was always thankful for this and at times a little ashamed. I was nowhere near as informed as Lisa, although all that changed when she moved into our home. I had to be on my game. Even then Lisa would double and triple check.

Each of the surgeons, oncologists, radiologists and palliative doctors we dealt with always went above and beyond for Lisa. The fact that she was in her early thirties and had such a determination to beat this disease, and such a love for life, spurred them on to try treatments that had shown even the slightest possibility of eradicating or shrinking Lisa's tumours.

It's quite common in Australia to go to your local medical centre and see whoever is available. But I'm glad that Lisa had stuck to one GP for all her care. Dealing with one GP as a family was great as they fully understood what everyone was going through. They made it their business to keep a close eye on all the family. When it came to GPs, we could not have asked for a better doctor. It didn't matter what symptoms Lisa was having, our GP wouldn't stop until she had something that worked. She would come

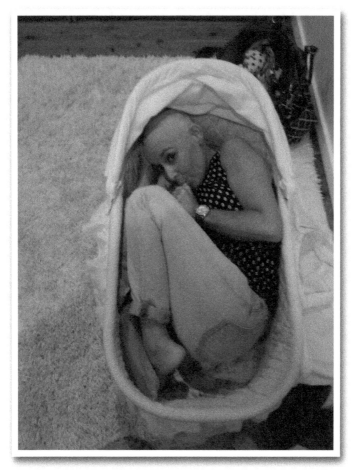

December 2013
Lisa trying out her niece Ava's bassinet. Even during the
toughest of times Lisa would find humour.

to our home, plump herself on the floor, and spend time talking to Lisa and the family about whatever was going on at the time. I would go as far as to say she was the glue that held us all together at times – the link in the chain between us and the specialists. We were blessed to have her on our team.

Hospital – My Home Away from Home

21/04/2016

We've been dealing with the C-word for four years now, and for two-and-a-half of those years I have been terminal. So as you can imagine, hospitals have become a regular fixture in my life. So much so that when I'm not at home, my niece Ava says, "Lisa's at the doctor's/hospital to make her belly better". And even when I'm on holiday or out with girlfriends, she just presumes that if I'm not at home, I'm somewhere getting treatment for my sore belly.

Nobody enjoys going to hospital. It's a cold, sterile place for sick, infectious people. I've been in the emergency department more these last few years than I've been in a supermarket.

Luckily for me, I rarely have to wait in the waiting room. If I haven't been taken by ambulance, once I or whoever is attending with me approaches triage (depending on if I am in too much pain to stand or talk), I'm then put in a wheelchair and escorted straight to a bed in the Emergency Department (ED).

I have had a few horrible experiences with people in triage who should NOT be in the industry of caring for people. I've had one nurse yell at us for having my brother and his wife sitting in the ED waiting room for me. I mean, seriously, why would my brother and sister-in-law want to wait for me? I mean, who cares that their sister has terminal cancer and every time she presents to ED there's the risk that this could be the tumour bleed that means she leaves hospital in a hearse? Who cares that this could be the time that her blood pressure drops so low that she becomes unconscious and becomes a vegetable?

I have no issue that the nurse wanted more seats available for sick people in the emergency department. It's all in the delivery. Simply ask them to relocate to the hospital café, or just ask them to move so that a potential patient can take the seat. I understand people have stressful days. But this was my second interaction with this woman, and on both occasions, I was made to feel that I was a burden rather than a patient.

I have absolutely no desire to be in the ED. I'd rather be at home watching *The Real Housewives of Goulburn* than be in hospital. I don't turn up to the hospital just for the fun of it. In fact, 90 per cent of the time I'm forced by my GP or a loved one to go there. I've usually been rolling around in excruciating can't-breathe-can't-talk-can't-walk-and-can't-cry pain. It's so painful yet I've still rejected everyone's demands to go to hospital. So, to have a nurse (whose role description states they support recovery by using care plans, carrying out care procedures and assessments, and evaluating and focusing on the needs of the patient rather than the illness or condition) make a patient feel like they are a nuisance is completely opposite to what they are actually meant to be doing.

Usually when I reach a bed in ED, I'm cannulated. (Though I can no longer be cannulated as all my veins have collapsed due to the amount of chemo I've had.) Thankfully, I now have a port in my chest where they put my cannula. A doctor then visits and assesses the situation, and any scans, bloods and so on that he/she feels are needed are ordered. Once all of these have been performed the doctor then determines whether I require hospital admission.

On my most recent visit on Friday the 15th of April, I woke up at 7am. It was about 25 degrees Celsius and I was freezing, shaking from head to toe. I took my temp and it was only 37.5 degrees Celsius. But because I was having rigors (all over body shakes), my dad drove me to the hospital. They admitted me straight away and took my temp. It was 40.9 degrees, very high, and my blood pressure was very low. They immediately put me on IV antibiotics and IV fluids. After a few hours, the doctor came in and told me that they were moving me to a different room with a view. But what he was actually doing was taking me to the resuscitation room because my blood pressure was so low it was considered almost fatal.

The doctor looked at me (Dad was sitting to my left) and he simply said, "Lisa, you are very sick, and I'd say it's the sickest you've ever been".

I responded by saying that once I was told that I wouldn't make it through the night. "Are we talking as bad as that?"

He replied, "You are very sick". That was enough for my Dad. He burst into tears and ran out of the room. I must admit that upon hearing that I didn't cry. I suppose I just went numb. I just thought, *No, I don't feel sick enough to be dying.*

The doctors and nurses were amazing. Two of them went out and consoled my dad, and luckily a girlfriend of mine came directly to the hospital to help comfort him.

> Nurses are the oxygen that keeps the hospital breathing.

Let me just say, on the whole nurses are amazing. They are not just the backbone of the health system, they are the tibia, the funny bone, the brains, the heart. They are the oxygen that keeps the hospital breathing. Nurses do not get enough credit. They are selfless human beings who get vomited on, spat at, sworn at, punched and so on. They are the ones who are on the frontline on a Friday night when you and your girlfriends decide it would be fun to do Jägerbombs or Fireball shots and throw in an ecstasy tablet or two. When you are rendered unconscious and choking on your own vomit, they treat you with the same respect that they treat the poor 80-year-old-woman who has come in with a broken hip. Because that's what nurses do. They care for you, no matter your social status, your race, your sex. If you haven't had a shower in a week and your body odour makes Pepé Le Pew smell like Chanel No.5, they still hold your hair while you vomit your spleen up, all because you thought it would be a good laugh to get wasted. And they do this for nowhere near enough pay!

So back to Friday.

I was transferred to ICU at the private hospital and was greeted by the nurse on duty. It all started to go downhill from there. As soon as I was transferred to the bed, I could tell it was one of those air mattresses that constantly move so that you don't get bed sores. The problem is these mattresses cause me major nerve pain from my tumours and have caused my readmission to hospital before. So I immediately asked if she could order a normal mattress.

She replied loudly and aggressively, "That will not be happening tonight. I'll turn the mattress off and the nurse in the morning will sort that out. I've got other things to do that are more important than ordering you a new mattress". I have to admit I cried. It was 9pm, and it had been a long, scary day. I hadn't eaten or drunk, and I was vulnerable. My dad was made to stay outside at this point. She then turned the mattress off. It deflated and left what I can only describe as speed humps all over the flat bed. I was expected to sleep on that when I was already in pain.

So I bit my tongue. She then proceeded to give me an ECG. Without any warning, she pulled my gown right up, exposing my whole naked body while the blinds were open. I politely asked her to close the blinds, to which she responded, "Don't tell me you're shy". It all just got worse from there.

I accidentally knocked one of the little clips for the ECG off, and she yelled at me for that too. After that my dad was allowed in. The first thing he mentioned was the piss poor excuse for a mattress I was sitting on. That was it. She turned around and yelled at him too. I could see the rage in my dad's face, like the old cartoons where their face goes beetroot red and steam shoots from their ears. I just looked at him with those pleading eyes. *Pleeeeease don't say anything. I have to spend ten more hours with this person alone.* So he didn't say anything. He was then overly nice to her in the hope that she would become nicer. But no, that didn't work.

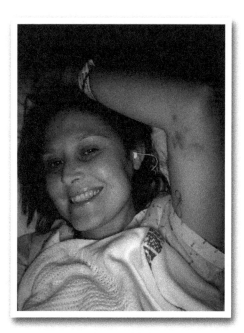

16 April 2016
Lisa at Greenslopes Private Hospital in Brisbane. Another hospital stay and another late-night selfie.

This sort of thing just kept on happening but with other nurses coming in and just naturally doing the right thing. One nurse saw my deflated mattress and immediately ordered me a new one. It got left outside my room, though, until the nurse looking after me could be bothered sorting it out. She sat at her desk flicking through a *Who* magazine for that whole time – her way of showing me who's in control.

I also was hooked up to a bunch of machines and was not allowed to walk far due to my low blood pressure. But because of my pelvic tumours I need to pee a lot, and I had to use the commode. When I finished, I asked her if she could leave it there as I pee regularly. That was too hard. Once again, another nurse came in and suggested that we leave the commode in the room. I then fell asleep, woke up and it was gone again. I was also told that this nurse wasn't a butler when I asked her to please pass me one of my bags that I couldn't reach. Seriously, I love nurses and feel that they do a fantastic job in a situation I wouldn't choose. But this was unbearable.

I was then transferred to the cancer ward where I had numerous nurses, and they were all fabulous. I spent only three days in there as the adrenalin through my IV had increased my blood pressure and the IV antibiotics had started to clear up the pneumonia in my lungs and the septicaemia in my blood. The great thing about being palliative is that the doctors and nurses try to get you fit enough to be out of hospital as quickly as possible, as they know how much time you spend in them.

I have been admitted to hospital so many times, I couldn't tell you the exact number. And although you never want to be there, I have to say that my overall experience with the numerous hospitals, nurses and doctors has been really good. My advice would be that you are called a patient for that exact reason. You need to be patient. You are not the only person there being treated. For every one of you, there is someone else worse off. Give the nurses and doctors a break. They are trying their best. I'm not saying they're all fabulous, but you just have to be reasonable. If you feel you're not being appropriately attended to, let them know. They're not mind readers; just speak up.

I only hope, for whoever is reading this, that you never have to go through what I go through regularly. Going to hospital once is not fun, never mind every few weeks.

> Don't use hospital as a medical centre or a GP.

My parting words would be: Don't use hospital as a medical centre or a GP. If you have a cold or an ingrown toe nail, go to the doctor not

ED. If you are truly sick, go to the hospital. The Emergency Department is already bursting at the seams, so use your common sense and only present to the ED if you need to.

How I Really Feel

24/04/2016

This will probably be the most honest blog I've written to date. In fact, it may be the most honest I've been with myself.

It's 1.20am. As I lie here with liver pain and regurgitating my dinner, I'm scared. I'm really scared. I can feel a tumour in the centre of my upper abdomen, the one I felt when it first returned. After radiation I have no other option. Even if I did, let's be honest, I've tried the best of the best: immunotherapies, chemotherapies and kinase inhibitors. It probably won't work. I'm not being a defeatist, and I can hear my friends out there saying, "Come on, Lisa. This isn't you. Where's that positive Lisa? The one who has beat it every time. They told her she wouldn't, well she's still here!"

I've always had these doubts and I've still managed to get through. I just haven't always told you when I feel this way.

I think we (those with cancer) often spend more of our energy protecting our loved ones from the reality that is cancer. We worry more about what you're worrying about than about ourselves. Well, I do anyway. I've often said that I'm glad it was me and not one of my family members or loved ones. And that's not being a martyr. I just don't think I could deal with it. I don't think I could watch them go through the pain and sickness that I have and not be able to make it better. Feeling helpless doesn't look good on me.

As I joke about sunbathing and saying things like, "Well, I've already got terminal cancer. I may as well die with a tan," the truth is I'm shitting myself. I'm not saying I'm scared all the time; most of the time I'm not. But there are moments like this – when the house is silent, I'm alone with my thoughts and I've had two shots of pain medication for my liver aching from the pressing tumours – that I could just burst into tears.

I have so many fears when it comes to dying, but my biggest would be 'FOMO': fear of missing out. When I die, I'm not going to be here any longer. I'm not going to be here to answer Rebecca's call when she wants to bitch about her long day at work. I'm probably not going to be there when Ava starts primary school or be there to explain why that boy on the bus keeps pulling her hair. Will I be around for the next series of *House of Cards*? (Yes, I'm being serious.) Will I be around for my friend Kieran's daughter's eighteenth? Will I still be around when my friend Sharon's house is built? Will this be my last Christmas or birthday? And the list goes on.

The thought of not being around scares the shit out of me. Yes, I want my family to be one of those families that sets a place at the dinner table for me on special occasions. I want Theresa Caputo to rock up to my parents' door and communicate with me from the other side. Better still I want to be a ghost/spirit. For family members' future reference, I will not appear to you in the bathroom/toilet. I will not appear in the bedroom. My choice of location will be a main living area and, if possible, I will knock three times before I appear, so you're not scared. I've discussed this with my brother and he has flat out refused a visit from me from the other side. So for you, Steven, I will just observe and not communicate. I will do that from any room in your house. I'm not even going to afford you the same privacy as those who want to see me. So if this bothers you, perhaps you may want to change your mind about seeing me when I visit from heaven. (Yeah, that's right. I'm pretty certain I'll get in.)

My biggest fear of them all is for my parents. You know how there's always one of the kids that will be the one to look after your parents when they get old? There's a sort of unspoken understanding? Well, I believe that was me, and to be quite honest, the thought of not being around to be their carer scares me. As much as I love my brother, will he be able to look after them the way I could? I'm sure he'll be totally fine, but it's just not the way it was meant to be.

Another stupid thought is: *Will many people turn up to my funeral?* I know, I know, I know. I've actually now realised that it doesn't really matter. I mean I'm not going to be there, unless something very wrong happens. But it still sneaks into my head sometimes. Then there's the logistics of it; New South

Wales or Queensland? I know I want to use my priest from the Central Coast, but as for where to have the funeral, I still can't decide.

What colour coffin? One thing for certain is I'm going to make sure the lining of my coffin or casket (yes, there is a difference) is not velvet. I can't stand the feeling of it, and dead or not I don't want it near me.

Flowers? NO LILIES. The slightest whiff and my nose runs faster than Usain Bolt. Once again, I know I'm dead and allergies don't matter anymore. But I don't care. White and green chrysanthemums are great. They're beautiful and they don't smell.

Who does the eulogy? What songs? Bury or cremate?

I originally wanted to be buried, but that opens a whole other can of worms like where to be buried. So for me the easiest option is to cremate. That way I don't need to decide where to be buried and my ashes can be separated and given to different loved ones. I've already spoken with my priest about whether separating ashes could cause issues with my soul and going to heaven. He advised me that your body is just a shell – a vessel. Once you die your spirit goes to heaven and any physical remains mean nothing. So it's totally acceptable to cremate and separate. (You see that? I'm sad and I'm still able to rhyme.)

I haven't felt like this since first finding out it was back. I look at old ladies and think, *You don't know how lucky you are*, especially when you hear them telling the cashier about their new hearing aid not working properly and how life is so hard. I get it. Your joints ache, and you can't see or hear properly anymore. But you're here to tell the story, and that's what matters.

I go to bed every night and repeat the same prayer: I ask God to spare me.

I beg Him/Her for a miracle and a cure, and every morning that I wake up I thank Him/Her for sparing me again. And then I get up and that good old grim reaper is still looking over my shoulder. I like to think that he and I have become mates and, maybe, that's why he's given me more time.

You never know what tomorrow may hold. Last Friday I was dying; this Friday I was painting dragons with my niece. Life really can change in the blink of an eye. So when you wake up tomorrow, embrace the new day, hug and kiss your loved ones, or ring them if you can't see them. Go to work and bitch and moan that the day will never end, but when it does, take a look at the sun going down and feel some appreciation. No matter what, the sun will still rise, and the sun will still set tomorrow. All those crappy, annoying things that happen in between are just that: crappy little annoyances. Life should be about sunsets not BoxSets. Get out there and take in its beauty. We are blessed every day to breathe in the beauty that is our world.

> We are blessed every day to breathe in the beauty that is our world.

I've written this blog over a couple of days, and as we speak, I am sitting with the sun shining and it's a balmy 27 degrees Celsius in autumn. While most people are out having a lovely Sunday drive with their loved ones or significant other, appreciating the day for what it is, I am appreciating it because I'm sitting here able to type, alive. Last night I went to bed scared that I may not wake up.

There are many things that come to mind when I think of Lisa's cancer journey, her excruciating pain being first and foremost. But this is closely followed by her fear.

Fear of going into the hospital and not getting out.

Fear of being under difficult nurses' care again. (It's sad how one very nasty experience can overshadow the many wonderful nursing experiences Lisa had experienced.)

Fear of Ava growing up without her and forgetting the beautiful memories they had made.

Lisa's biggest fear was of death itself.

Unfortunately, this was one of those times that reading Google only heightened Lisa's fear. The thought of the unbearable pain, and of not being able to breathe, terrified her. Lisa tried to hide her fear from us for a very long time. But her face had 'fear' written all over it with each trip to the ER.

I know that Lisa blamed steroids for her inability to get to sleep, and they definitely didn't help, but I truly believe Lisa was frightened she wouldn't wake up. For her last six months, Lisa couldn't sleep lying down as she would regurgitate in her sleep and could easily choke. Tumour pain and troubled breathing also made it difficult to sleep lying down. We would try and prop her up and make her comfortable with additional pillows and cushions, but even when we managed to get her comfortable, she would put Netflix on or start writing a blog, just to keep her mind busy and avoid sleep.

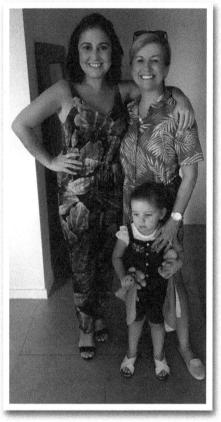

25 April 2016
Lisa, Geraldine and Ava at home before a day out. Her strength never failed to amaze us.

We would watch her trail her body around the house, exhausted from all it had been through. But her head and heart were strong. It was the most heart-breaking thing I've ever seen, and I prayed that God would let Lisa slip away in her sleep. Life should never be so hard and so cruel.

Although Lisa declined therapy, I definitely needed it. As the disease spread and the pain continued to get worse, so would the tears I'd cry at counselling. It was the one place I didn't have to be strong and I didn't have to pretend. I was sad, I was angry, and I was frightened – like Lisa. As bad as it sounds, I don't know what frightened me most – the thought of

Lisa passing or the thought of Lisa living with this cruel disease. And that's where guilt replaced all other feelings. How could a mother wish her own daughter dead? It's not until you live through the alternative that you will ever understand how this could be. Lisa was fighting for every day, every minute and every second. But it came at a cost and she paid a very high price. Her strength and determination never failed to surprise me.

> Her strength and determination never failed to surprise me.

Dating While You're Dying

01/05/2016

If Bridget Jones thought she had issues dating, imagine dating when you have terminal cancer. I have the same issues Bridget had: that bee-stung bloated face (although I think that's more Renée Zellweger's face than character acting), granny undies that way outweigh lacy Victoria's Secret underwear in my drawer, wine as my main form of hydration and I suffer from chronic verbal diarrhoea. If there's something inappropriate to be said, I am the one who will say it. Just ask any of my friends or family. I have no filter, and nor do I intend to start filtering what I say. Stuff it, I have terminal cancer. If I want to say something, I'll say it and deal with the nuclear fallout later.

I am a 34-year-old woman who has recently separated from my long-term partner of nearly 14 years. I say recently, but really it was June last year. But we've continued to communicate since maybe eight weeks after breaking up.

Breaking up was a difficult decision to make. He and I had been together since I was 19 turning 20. He came into my life at a very uncertain time for me. My parents and brother were moving back to Ireland and I was moving out of home for the first time. I had to become an adult overnight. I mean I had done laundry, cooked dinners and washed dishes, but I'd never had to pay for my clothes that I had to wash. I never had to pay for the steak that I cooked, and I certainly never had to pay for the electricity or water usage to do the dishes. So I suppose you could say I met my ex-partner at a time that I was confused and very unsure about my future.

He was suave, had a secure job and a quirky/wicked sense of humour, and he made my heart jump and my face turn red when I saw him. But there was one thing most people noticed first: he was older. And when I say older, I mean a LOT older. And if I'm honest, he brought more baggage with him than Kim Kardashian would on a one-week trip to New York Fashion Week. But I fell in love. I loved his confidence, which I would probably now categorise as ego.

Anyway I'm not going to get into the ups, downs and sideways of our long, long, long relationship. But I can say, for all our faults, from the time I was initially diagnosed with cancer and the time I was told it had come back, he

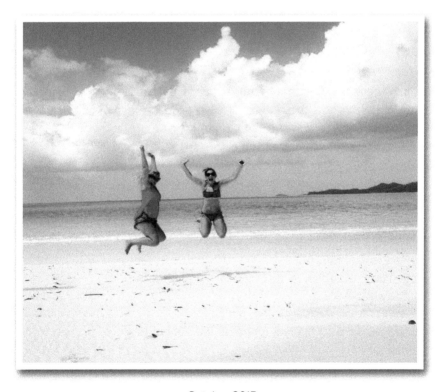

October 2015
Aleana McGuiness and Lisa at the Whitsundays enjoying a day at
the beach four months after Lisa's break-up with her partner.

was there, by my side, at every moment for every meeting, every treatment, every surgery, every toxic vomit. When my hair started to fall out, we shared the hair shaving duties with his electric razor. He was the one who would make my gluten-free bacon and egg rolls when I was on chemo at any hour of the night. If I wanted it at 3.30am he would get up and do it. So I could never complain or say a bad word about his commitment to caring for me while I was sick. Sadly, though, he and I just didn't work cohesively as a couple. When the cancer came initially, we were actually at a crossroads. Let's just say that when this ugly C-word raised its head, we were already in an unstable position. But I got cancer and those other problems got swept under the rug.

Today I have absolutely no desire to be in a relationship. I don't know if it's because of my break-up or because my libido is non-existent due to my hormones being everywhere from the myriad of treatments I've had. But I can honestly say that a relationship, a quickie in a Best Western, a swipe right on Tinder or a drunken kiss in a nightclub are absolutely the last things on my mind.

I know there are many men and women who have a chronic illness or terminal disease out there that still have a desire to love and be loved. I'm just not one of them. Well, at the moment I'm not, and I often wonder if I was, how one would broach the subject. So, you're at a bar and a guy approaches you and asks to buy you a drink. Do you blurt it out mid drink invitation? Do you wait until after your first sip? Do you wait until you're finished the drink, or do you wait until you're three sheets to the wind and then admit that you're expiring as you speak? Or just not tell them at all? What is the terminal disease admission etiquette? Just like you single mothers and fathers out there, I'm sure you've all grappled with the 'When do you drop the I-have-a-kid bomb?'

I'm sure diving back into the dating pool at my age already has its challenges. Like for me, I suppose if the cancer didn't exist, men would probably be thinking, *Why? Why are you still single at this age? Haven't you been married by now, at least once? Don't you have a kid? What's wrong with you that you've reached your mid-thirties and no-one, NO-ONE has thought enough of you to at least get you pregnant?*

Then there's the old 'Are you married?' chestnut that you're inevitably asked when you're at treatment or admitted to hospital. Apparently, once you hit 30 it is abnormal to not be married or at least divorced. To be honest, even if I didn't have the Big C, I still think I would have broken up with my partner. I'd be in the same position but not dying.

I am obviously in the minority when it comes to wanting to be single and alone and not dating. All you have to do is look at the amount of dating sites on Google or dating site ads on TV and the fact that these dating websites are now sub-grouped and so specific, like Ashley Madison. Married, who cares?

- Looking for that likeminded Christian that wants to be chaste until your honeymoon? Go to chrisitianconnection.com.
- Love your dog like they're your daughter and not your pet? Why not go to animalpeople.com?
- Are you tall and looking for that equally vertically unchallenged soulmate? Go to tallfriends.com.

Here are two more, and I must admit they're my favourite of the most specific dating sites. They're so good I can't decide which one wins the 'most uniquely unambiguous of all dating sites ever created'.

- If you're into 'furry fandom', dressing up and behaving like an animal of some sort, fear not. Your perfect furry friend is waiting for you at furrymate.com
- Or for those of you who really are big kids at heart and love wearing nappies, don't despair. You too can also find your nappy wearing soulmate at diapermates.com.

Whatever happened to plain old RSVP where you find out that the guy you've met online has a diaper fetish the traditional way, by snooping through his wardrobes when he's popped out to pick up your Chinese takeaway? I mean, have we become that lazy that we can't even do our own vetting? People, finding out these wonder things about the person you're dating is half the fun of dating!

I suppose if the guy doesn't want a long-term thing then I might be in with a chance, what with my rapidly approaching expiration date and all. For now

Note to self: Copyright 'Terminal Tinder'.

I'm happy the way things are: just me, myself and I. Eventually when someone has created 'Terminal Tinder' (Note to self: Copyright 'Terminal Tinder'), maybe I'll be ready to swipe right. But will someone swipe right for me?

When Peter and I were on our way to Ireland to live for a few years, when Lisa was 19, we had a stopover in Singapore for a few days. As we were walking around sightseeing, I had this empty feeling like I'd left my purse at home. I couldn't shake it. In reality, I hadn't forgotten something. It was our daughter that was missing, and it was extremely difficult to understand.

Now, I look back at that time and all I can think is: *If only we knew then what we know now.* We wasted precious time without our girl. As far as we were concerned it was the best time for us to go. We would be back in a few years and fully expected that, by that time, Lisa would have met the man of her dreams. We could plan a beautiful wedding together and she'd have her happy-ever-after. But unfortunately, life doesn't always give you the fairy-tale ending.

As much as Lisa's relationship with her partner was difficult for us to accept, he was there when it mattered. But unfortunately it came at a cost. Thankfully, once the relationship had ended, it didn't take Lisa long to realise she had done the right thing. The only person she had to worry about going forward was herself.

As Lisa has mentioned, she was happy being single, though she continued to struggle with her everchanging appearance. However, it didn't stop guys looking at her when we were out. Someone always approached her and struck up a conversation. But because Lisa wasn't happy with how she looked, she failed to see that others still found her attractive. This made me so sad because I just wanted her to see what we – her family, friends and even strangers – saw when we looked at her: a beautiful 34-year-old woman with a vibrant personality to match.

Although Lisa wasn't ever the type of girl that longed for the fairy-tale wedding, I think that as her health deteriorated, she secretly entertained the thought of having a wedding day before she passed. Male friends had suggested this to Lisa. Although she declined at the time, if she'd had a bit longer maybe she would have taken one of the guys up on their offer. It saddens me to think of her missing out on that special day, with her dad never getting the chance to walk her down the aisle. But then I remember all the special times we got to spend together, and the truth is not a lot of families get these opportunities. We did make the most of every opportunity and our mantra 'no regrets', which I still live by.

Why Me Day

06/05/2016

Today has been hard. Today has been scary. Today has been the day from hell.

Today is not unique. I have had days like this before, maybe in a different state in a different doctor's office. But the message was exactly the same: "The treatment has not worked. Your tumours have grown and there's not really anywhere we can go from here."

When I was first told my cancer was back, in September 2013, I was told I'd have weeks, maybe months, to live. So I did what any sensible human being does upon hearing this news. I ignored it. No, I didn't ignore the fact that my cancer was back and that it was terminal. But I ignored the weeks or months part. And for the most part that's worked for me. Since my cancer's return, no treatment has ever really worked. But it's maybe given me a month here or there, and those months add up after a while.

> The treatment has not worked.

In between now and then, if you've read my previous blogs you would know I've tried numerous therapies and surgeries. Each one gave us a little hope for a little while, but inevitably my army of tumours would march themselves back into my body and begin to invade again.

November 2014 was the biggest fright of all.

I had been in hospital that week with a suspected tumour bleed. On the day of my return home from hospital, I was still experiencing pain, but it was bearable. I remember walking from the lounge room to my bedroom. I was slouching from the pain, and then it hit like a thousand shards of hot molten glass to my upper abdomen. I fell to the bedroom floor trying to scream, but I couldn't from the sheer agony of what my body was going through. I couldn't breathe from the pain. My partner and mum rushed to help me, but they could tell there was nothing they could do. They had to call the ambulance.

I don't know how long it took for the ambulance to arrive, but if it was ten minutes it felt like ten hours. The paramedics rushed into the bedroom and immediately cannulated me and started pumping the morphine in. But nothing would improve my pain levels. They then discussed whether to administer ketamine (a drug commonly used by doctors or veterinarians as an anaesthetic). Luckily for me my cancer type didn't allow me to have this drug. For those of you who don't know me personally, I am barely 5-foot-tall, and at the time I was only about 40 kilograms (88 pounds). So it didn't take much morphine to send me into a very sleepy state. But they kept pumping the stuff into me.

By the time I arrived at the hospital, I was still in enormous pain even though I'd had enough morphine in my system to knock an entire football team out. Next thing I remember was everyone rallying around me, calling out my name. That was the time I nearly died. I had so much morphine in my system that I had overdosed. I was told my eyes rolled into the back of my head and that was it. But I came back around.

That night my left foot stopped working because of my pelvic tumours pressing on nerves. At one point I tried to stand up and just fell to the ground. My bladder stopped working for the same reason. I just remember being hunched up in a ball in a hospital room with friends and family members coming from all over the place, at all hours of the night. I kept asking if I was dying, and nobody would say yes. That was, of course, if they could understand my incoherent babble from the amount of morphine in my system.

I would start weird conversations in my head and answer myself out loud, much to the fear of those around me. I'm sure that under any normal circumstances, my behaviour would have been recorded and submitted to *The Ellen Show*. But because of the seriousness of the situation, we couldn't enjoy the comedy gold that was the one-woman act for one night only: the Lisa's-Dying-But-Geez-She's-Funny-on-Morphine Show. We can look back now and have a laugh. I just wish someone had the foresight to record it, stuff time and a place, for future reference. If I am ever high on any pain meds like that again, pull that phone out and hit record. I wanna see that shit!

That night was a long one; that weekend was even longer. I had radiation for the first time, to try to stop my tumour bleed, not to reduce tumour size. It was simply a palliative measure. I didn't know it at the time, but the doctors didn't think I'd make it through that night. Then they didn't think I'd make it through the weekend. They even brought the priest in, but I rallied and was visited by palliative nurses who told me I probably wouldn't see another Christmas. (We were in November.) Considering the date on this, you obviously know I made it to Christmas that year and the one after that. For some reason my tumours reacted to the radiation. Some died and others shrunk, and my overall disease reduced dramatically.

I've had a few other occasions, now and then, where I've been told weeks not months. But each time I manage to pull a little miracle out of my arse.

Leading up to this recent scan, I've been experiencing more pain. I've also been regurgitating a lot of my food, which means some of my stomach tumours have grown and are starting to cause blockages. So I sort of had a bad feeling that the news I was going to receive today wasn't going to be fabulous. But you're never quite prepared to hear those words. No matter how many times I've heard them before, it always feels like the first time.

The poor oncologist delivering the deadly blow often doesn't quite know where to look, or is it me that doesn't quite know where to look? Sort of like that awkward stage when you like a guy and you both do that coy I'm-looking-at-you-not-really-but-I-am-looking-at-you look. You know the one. Well, when an oncologist is telling you that things don't look great, it's kind of like that.

Today, there was my oncologist, me and my mum in the room. My mum was sitting to the left and slightly behind me, so out of eye contact. My oncologist was sitting in front of me. But when he's delivering the things-aren't-looking-great speech, it's as if we're all in different corners of the globe. We're in the same small office, but we can't feel any further away from each other. I look in every direction: up, down, sideways, peek at mum, tap the desk, play with my oncologist's mousepad. I look everywhere but in anybody's eyes, because if I have direct eye contact, I might just break down. And I can't do that. I can't let myself cry. I've cried too many tears over this bastard already.

> I can't let myself cry. I've cried too many tears over this bastard already.

I also wore mascara today that isn't waterproof, so I couldn't let it happen.

I often wonder if doctors have to take a class on how to inform a patient that they're dying. Do they actually feel anything when they're saying it? If they do feel sad, does it ever get any easier? We spend so much time thinking about ourselves and how we react to hearing the words, we forget that there's a whole other human being on the other side of the desk delivering the death blow.

The car ride home is never fun either. Mum and I get in the car and we sort of debrief and each give the other our version of what we think was said in the meeting. Even though you're in the same room, hearing the same words, you will always have a difference of opinion as to what was said. It's funny how human beings can comprehend the exact same words completely differently. I'll tell Mum she needs to let me have the shits at the situation for a while. I'll say the f-word, followed by the c-word (yep carrot), followed by the f-word again, and so on. Then I'll start to make my phone calls to people, informing them of the shit news, and I'll say it all pretty matter-of-factly. I'll tell them I'm not in the mood to talk about it yet, and by that point I'm home.

We went and watched a movie after the news today, and I was into it for about the first hour. But after that it's a blur.

The rest of today was a series of numb, strange exchanges with tonnes of people messaging or calling. I know they care, and that's lovely, but I never feel like talking the 'day of'. Today is a blur. I look at random people.

Why me and not you? You're watching the same movie as me and the biggest worry you have is where you'll have dinner after it. Meanwhile I'm sitting here trying to digest the fact that I'm dying again. No shrinkage this time. Not stable disease. No little miracle pulled out of my arse. No, this time I have to face the reality again of what 'terminal' actually means.

What's so special about you that you get to live while I don't? Why me?

I don't ask why me very often, and tomorrow I'll regret that I even let myself go there, even if it was just for a minute. But today

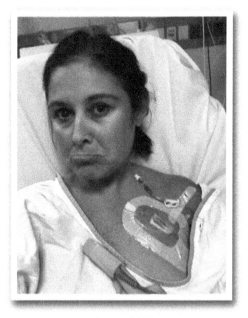

10 May 2016
Lisa at the PA Hospital, Brisbane, during another emergency hospital visit.

is a *Why Me?* day, and I suppose we're all entitled to one every now and then.

I Don't Want to Be in a Better Place

13/05/2016

So, it's been over a week since I found out that the radiation didn't work this time and the words "You should have died when you were last admitted to hospital" came out of my oncologist's mouth. Fast forward to now and here I am in palliative care, barely able to breathe due to the pain from my liver tumours pressing on my diaphragm.

We have changed my meds once again, and the one thing I desperately want to go away is the inability to breathe properly. I am begging all the gods to take this and my liver pain away. But when do I come to the point of acceptance? When do things get so bad that I finally let it take me?

Writing this now makes me want to sob, uncontrollably. People say "You'll be in a better place, pain free. We're the ones left behind, having to deal with getting our heads all around this". Well, you know what? I don't wanna be in a better place. I like right where I am, thank you. Well, not in palliative care at the hospital, but when I'm at home, playing with my niece or making dinner. I really love those simple things.

I'm not ready. I AM NOT READY!!!! YOU stare death in the face and see how you feel.

As I sit here typing this blog, yet another sobbing relative has retreated to the palliative ward hallway. Are they crying from fear? Are they crying from seeing their loved one in so much pain? Or are they crying because their loved one has finally passed?

What do I do? I put my headphones on and turn the music up. Well, what else do I do? Do I sit and listen to their pain and make myself feel worse? (Yes, I know. It's not about me. A poor family has just lost their loved one and I'm trying to protect myself.) Or do I listen and let their fear and sadness consume me and, in turn, make me even more scared?

I choose to drown it out. I'm sorry if that's cold, but I just can't deal with the reality of it all. So I do understand that, for those left behind, it is incredibly hard. And I understand why they would think that it's harder on them than it is on me.

But imagine not being around.

Imagine not being there for the little things in life, never mind the big things.

Basically, this whole 'SHITuation' is exactly that: shit!

I still can't believe that the immunotherapy I spent $7000 on every three weeks for four times has wrecked my lungs, and that it could quite possibly be my lungs that kill me, not the actual cancer! So I'm pissed off. I'm pissed off that I actually paid for the possibility of an earlier demise. I paid for this shit to be injected into my veins, and it not only damaged my lungs, it also

> Basically, this whole 'SHITuation' is exactly that: shit!

116

made my tumours grow faster and larger! Yes, I'm resenting it, and I know if I hadn't done it, I would have always asked 'what if?' So I had to do it.

I also don't want to dissuade people from trying anything they can. The drug I was on is an amazing drug with proven results. But for me, sadly, I feel it has increased my tumour growth rate and size. The old you're-damned-if-you-do-and-you're-damned-if-you-don't situation.

I had a meeting with the palliative doctor yesterday (not my regular oncologist). He basically said my disease had progressed 'rapidly' – another frightening word. I then rang my oncologist and asked him, and he said the same thing except he used the words 'This is shit'. There's that word again. They should change the word 'cancer' to 'shit'!

I'm not ready yet. I don't want to go. No matter how much fun it is on the other side (and the thought of partying with both Prince and Princess Diana at the same time thrills me), I'd still rather be playing dolls with my niece down here on earth in our little lounge room.

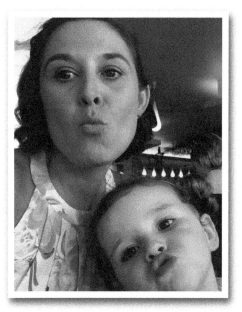

20 November 2015
Lisa and Ava's selfie pout
during a trip into Brisbane.

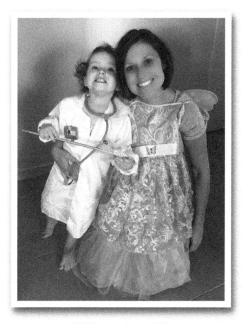

30 December 2015
Lisa and Ava at home playing dress-up.

I want to thank you all for your love and support, and I am hoping and praying that you will all be reading another blog from me soon.

Stay fabulous, people. X

As parents, we should always know what to say when our kids are hurting or are in danger. But the reality is we don't. We've probably never watched our child suffer to the point where you can practically feel their pain, so how in hell's name are we meant to know the right thing to say? We can't reassure them by telling them it'll all be all right ... because it won't

The comment Lisa mentions about being in a better place more than likely came from me. I have read all the cancer books that tell you your loved one is hanging on for you, waiting for you to tell them it's okay to go. But in our case, it wasn't as straight forward. Lisa proved time and time again that she would endure whatever was thrown at her and would never throw in the towel. I was really struggling at this stage. Lisa was so ill, I didn't see how she could take anymore. Peter was somewhat in denial. He wanted her to live so much that he couldn't even think about her dying, and at times he wouldn't even discuss it. But when all was said and done, someone needed to try and ease Lisa's fear of death. Someone needed to let her know that she had fought long and hard and it was okay to rest. And that someone was me.

As expected, and as Lisa has verbalised in her blog, the conversation was blanked. Lisa wasn't ready to go and continued to fight for all she was worth.

> Lisa wasn't ready to go and continued to fight.

As much as Lisa was feeling she had lost complete control of every aspect of her life, she was still the driving force throughout her cancer journey. The medical experts could make suggestions and recommendations based on the facts put in front of them, but when push came to shove, Lisa was the decision maker every step of the way, as it should be.

I sat in many meetings with Lisa and different members of her medical team. I saw that they would quite often agree to give any treatment or medication Lisa suggested a go because of her determination and desperation to live as long as she could – despite their hesitancy if they were not confident of the impact and outcome.

I worried about how we would prepare Lisa for passing if she continued to believe that there was another lifeline.

Just to be clear, Lisa's suggestions were not life-threating. But at times they were quite left of field. Even when radiation had minimal impact on Lisa's condition, she practically begged for another round just to be sure.

Urinary Catheter – A Necessary Evil with Good Intentions

16/05/2016

A Light-Hearted Blog for a Heavy-Hearted Week

Aahh the urinary catheter. Just sounds convenient, doesn't it? The answer to every lazy man/woman's dreams. The answer to every busy mum who's running around not having the luxury of 30 seconds to sit on the porcelain throne and pee without interruption. Imagine never having to pause your favourite TV show again for a pesky pee break. Peeing. It takes up so much time!

Say you urinate the average seven times a day, and say you take 30 seconds each time you go. (This is solely for urination purposes. I am not going to get into the mysteries that are the bowels tonight. Well, I haven't planned to, but who knows where this blog could take us?) That works out to be a total of about 1273.3333 minutes over 365 days. If you live to, say, 78, that's a total of about 99,319.9974 minutes wasted hovering over a toilet or a urinal, behind a bush, in a pool or wherever else you like to relieve yourself. Believe me, I'm not here to judge, unless it's illegal. Well, then I'm going to judge you, as you should be judged.

So having this wonderful time-saving device inserted into your urethra is one of the few medical procedures I feel that maybe a man would find a tad more uncomfortable than a woman. I mean, honestly, it's not a pleasant thought, is it? To have something foreign shoved up that tiny little hole? I bet you're all squeezing your knees together as you read. Steven (my brother), I can just imagine the face you're pulling in disgust at the lack of gentility and etiquette in relation to this matter. Ah well, it is what it is. It all sounds like a land of unicorns and leprechauns, doesn't it? Yes, there is the downside that you have to haul a bag of your pee around for all to judge your water intake. In reality, a piece of plastic tubing shoved up your fanny with a balloon on the end (to keep it from falling out) is painful and uncomfortable and just asking for an infection.

The first time you get a catheter in while you're awake is a bit daunting. The awkwardness of having a nurse stare up your hoo haa is never a nice thought, but it is a necessary evil in some hospital admissions. Believe me, if you've just gone through a ten-hour abdominal surgery, you'll be glad you don't have to get up and go to the toilet. But they're not the ones I'm talking about. I'm talking about the ones you get when you're awake.

I sadly have had more urinary catheters than I would like to admit, but I promised you warts and all in this blog. My main reason for getting them now is because of the size of my bladder tumours. They are causing blockages and putting pressure on the neck of my bladder, so I can't 'go' properly or sometimes at all.

In all honesty, the whole process, if done correctly, is very easy and not too uncomfortable at all, unless they do it wrong. I, my friends, have had it done wrong and it's a dark, dark 48 hours that I would rather not revisit. EVER!

I'm not going to go into a blow-by-blow account of how they insert it. I'm not a medical dictionary and I feel my description would not be totally correct. And let's be honest, it would probably be a bit biased, which would be unfair to the poor catheter as it really does have its good uses.

My issue now is that, after about 72 hours of having a catheter in, it all starts to become uncomfortable, even traumatised. I've also had an incident that left my urethra traumatised. I knelt up on the bed on top of my catheter tube by accident and the whole thing yanked out. Let's just say I didn't walk or pee right for at least three days.

Catheters are sadly not natural to the body, so the body often rejects them by way of introducing infection to get rid of it. So the docs usually don't like leaving them in for extended periods anyway. Speaking of 'periods' ... Don't be alarmed if you're a woman and your period starts when you have a catheter inserted. It's actually quite common – just a fast fact for you.

I don't know how long this will stay in. The last I was told was indefinitely. Well, no thank you. I see your 'indefinitely' and raise it with a 'definitely'. I want it out and I want it out yesterday. It will be reviewed tomorrow by the palliative care doc, so we'll see what happens (fingers crossed).

So in short, catheters are certainly handy. They serve a great purpose. They don't hurt as much as you would imagine when you're getting it in or out. They pop the little balloon before taking it out and it slides right out. (I know, I know. TMI. Well, stop reading if it's too much for you lol.) They are a great little invention, just not a long-term one for me.

So sadly for those of you who feel a commercial catheter would be a god-send, I shall have to burst your catheter bubble (pun was definitely intended). I don't foresee Johnson & Johnson releasing the 'convenient catheter compact' any time soon.

So, to you my fellow *Terminally Fabulous* people, may you pee long and prosper. I'm keeping my fingers and toes crossed that my pee will one day again run free, just as nature intended it.

Love you peoples. Keep your chin up and your positivity coming. Thank you all for your love, support and guidance. Now go and have a nice long pee; you deserve one after all that.

> I'm keeping my fingers and toes crossed that my pee will one day again run free.

A Blog About the Bog

22/05/2016

If You Don't Like Toilet Humour, Don't Read This Blog About the Bog!

Bowels. We all have them, we all use them and we all don't like to talk about them. Or so you'd think. I talk about my bowels all day every day. Have I been? What was its consistency and colour? Small or big? You see, once you're diagnosed with cancer and start some treatment, whether curative or not, you will end up on some sort of drug that will bind you up tighter than a bondage scene from *Fifty Shades of Grey*.

Basically, steroids will clog you, anti-nausea meds will bung you and pain meds will block you up. Then there is the other myriad of drugs that cause your arse to pucker up like a dried raisin. Usually you're using a combination of all or some of these already arse-achingly blocking meds. So if you've been constipated, times that by 100 and you might just get an idea of how blocked one's plumbing becomes when sick with cancer. All the other shit that we put up with on a daily basis isn't enough, so let's just give her the shits but not let her shit!!!!!

Constipation is painful. It's like there is a boxing ring inside your stomach with ten fights going on simultaneously, all going 100 rounds. Then there's the constant heavy, bloated feeling that comes with it. It's just horrible. Unless you've had it, it's very hard to explain. My explanation is the best I could come up with at 12.45am on a Saturday night / Sunday morning.

Then there is the other side. Obviously, pain relief and treatment outrank constipation, so rather than reduce pain meds or change treatment for the cancer, you need to address the constipation. So the docs have to unclog you. You often end up in hospital in excruciating pain from constipation, and then you spend the next four or five days trying to crap. They will not discharge you until you poo. They will fill you full of Coloxyl drops (like drinking caramel flavoured cat's piss), Dulcolax drops, suppositories, enemas, Movicol and soooooo much more. Eventually, you are squirting liquid nitrogen out of your bunghole and you frequent the toilet more than any other room. Success ... apparently.

You don't get a happy medium or a happy ending. You are either one of two things: bunged up or flowing feverishly.

People don't realise how important it is to have a healthy relationship with your bowels. Remember, if you don't shit you die. So you've got to stay on top of that stuff.

> Remember, if you don't shit you die.

I say free the bowels. No longer should my predictive text change bowel to vowel when I type. (Even my iPhone has no respect for the bowels.) If you're lucky enough to have bowels that work, embrace it, feel privileged and be proud that you have been blessed with a working poo factory. Oh what I'd give to be the person who actually contemplates holding one in because they can't bear the thought of another human being walking into the bathroom mid-plop. I say we should not care about what other people think. I say unclench. Poo away. Let them plop and plop high!!!! Be proud. You are one lucky son of a bitch.

I am more inclined to be the person squatting there willing one out, to no avail. Either that or I'm running (well, walking at a decent pace or being pushed in my wheelchair) to the closest toilet because of my explosive diarrhoea.

What about those people who go at the same time every day like clockwork? How lucky are they? These are not unicorns; they do exist, and I know a couple of them. One in particular lives with me and could go ten times a day if they had the spare time in the day to actually crap that often. I'm jealous that shitting can come so easily to people and they often don't realise how lucky they are. Yes, I have a case of the brown-eyed monster!

So to those of you who are anally blessed, I salute you. I hope you never have to experience the pain or discomfort that is constipation, or the opposite that occurs upon trying to rectify it.

Let the plop run free. Wear it like a badge of honour. The next time you are in a public restroom and are lucky enough to be pooing, don't wait until the person next to you flushes or runs the tap or leaves the room. Do as I say and smile to yourself. Be proud that you are one of the chosen ones. You were given this wonderful gift, so use it and use it often!

Free the plop!

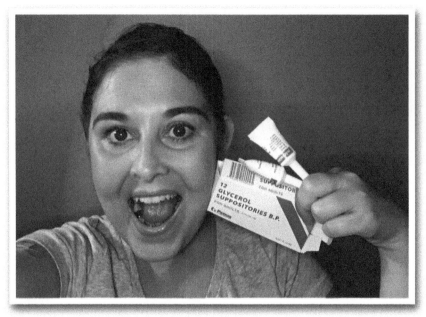

11 August 2016
Lisa with her suppositories! Blocked bowels were part of everyday life... a very painful part. Lisa had a never-ending list of medications to try to get some relief.

One thing I had to adjust to very quickly was how freely Lisa discussed her bowel movements. (And just to be very clear, I am not the ten times per day person in the house!) Poo regularity was discussed just like the daily weather. It didn't matter who was in the house; if there was an issue on that day, so be it. It was discussed.

I think initially Peter and I were quite embarrassed, but we soon learnt that discussing Lisa's poo was the least of our worries. The pain that came with constipation or a blockage was excruciating. There were many times when lying in bed we could hear Lisa crying with pain. Initially we would get up and offer her something to see if it would help, but she just wanted to be left alone. There was nothing anyone could do.

Coming Down from a Major Low – Isn't it Ironic?

26/05/2016

I've been home from hospital for a week now, and I am still trying to adapt to the new norm. Everybody gets excited about me coming home. You're in this huge hospital-escaping high and then reality hits like a giant clap of thunder right on your head: You're home. So why do you feel so blue?

The first few weeks at home after a decent hospital stay feels like you've just come off a two-week bender in Vegas, where you had unlimited money, alcohol and drug supply. When you get out, you have to realign yourself with your reality. You usually don't have the same amounts of drugs being constantly pumped into you, so you're coming down majorly. That's why I liken it to a bender. It's not because we play roulette at the nurses' station or we're slamming tequila shots at bedtime. And at home you just don't keep up with that same regimen (even if you're meant too ... oops).

It's physically and mentally draining. I feel like I'm an alien in my own home, walking around in a daze. Things don't feel real. I'm snappy, irrational, depressed, concerned and the list goes on. I also have to get my head around accepting that I actually did get out hospital after being basically told I would not make it out.

I was standing at the sink tonight, overlooking our lounge room, just watching everyone chatting and pottering about. My aunty and granny are over from Ireland, and I realised for the thousandth time that I'm not going to be here one day. This will all go on without me, whether I like it or not. Major FOMO and all they were doing was watching TV. Imagine if they were doing something interesting!

It's that reality check again. You see, I can ho hum about life when I'm not feeling major pain. But when you're admitted to hospital, it's that glaringly obvious reminder that you're dying. You see that word 'palliative' every day in the hallway and watch other people come into the ward only to leave with a sheet pulled over them and a butterfly placed on the empty room door. When people die in my palliative care ward, the nurses place a beautiful fake butterfly on the door.

To say that I'm harder to get along with after getting out of hospital is a complete understatement. I'm a total nutcase, just trying to get my mind and body around it.

> I'd say the mental stuff is harder to deal with.

Physically, you are also stuffed. You feel like you've ran a four-week marathon. Your muscles really deteriorate very quickly, and you don't tend to use them in hospital. You really only move from the bed to the toilet or down the hallway to the family area. So your body is in just as bad a shape as your mind. (Well, not quite. I'd say the mental stuff is harder to deal with.) Thankfully, my mum and the family have the patience of saints. They understand now and give me a wide berth.

My poor mum cops it all day long. I am a cantankerous bitch at the best of times, never mind when the chips are down. Then when I get out of hospital I am like a bear with a sore head all day. I don't know how she hasn't suffocated me in my sleep yet (death humour too soon?).

My mind and body are at war with each other. My mind says, "Get off your arse and do those dishes!" and my body says, "Get your dad to do them." You see I'm a doer. I do the dishes. I cook dinner. I do the laundry. I just like to do the do, and my stupid body doesn't allow me to do the do. Just let me do the goddamn do!!!! So today I did the do. I did laundry and I cooked dinner. That was a major feat. I know, give her a medal. She hung out some washing and baked a chook. A ten-year-old can do that. But for me who has had no energy or strength at all for the last few weeks, these little things are big things.

On top of getting out of hospital, the lady from palliative care came to my home to redo my advance health directive (AHD) the other day, for the third time. Apparently, the first and second times weren't traumatic enough. It's a laugh a minute!

For those of you who don't know what an AHD is, it is basically a piece of written document informing people of my medical intentions if I am incapable of doing so myself. It is signed and authenticated by a JP, but it can still be over-ruled. It's really more for the people who care about you, so there is no confusion. And it takes the stress out of making decisions, like if you should be put on a ventilator to help you breathe. That's a big decision to make, so if it's written down on a piece of paper, your mum, partner etcetera don't have to make that unenviable decision for you. It's also good information for the paramedics/ambulance officers, doctors and so on to have. If you have a terminal or chronic illness like me, they say you should leave it on top of the fridge and the paramedics know to look there.

This isn't just for terminally ill people or the elderly. Everyone should have an advance healthcare directive. God forbid you should have a serious car accident and you're unconscious, and when you arrive at hospital, you have a turn and stop breathing. Do they resuscitate or not?

Firstly, let me tell you, resuscitation is not like it is in the movies. It's not just compress-and-breathe. They have to compress your chest to 75 per cent, and it breaks your rib cage bones. I've been told by health professionals that you actually hear the bones breaking. Quite often you end up being ventilated, or you could be brain dead. Now for a healthy 34-year-old, with no other disease or illness, resuscitation is still an option for you. But for me, to go through all of that and then still be dying anyway, it makes no sense. So that's the reason I did my AHD for the third time today.

Confronting does not begin to describe it. Discussing and making decisions about these things is bloody hard, to say the least, especially when you're closer to your expiry date than most.

Do you want ventilation?
Do you want nutrition if you can't eat?
Do you want major surgery if needed?

And the list goes on.

You just have to sit there and suck it up whilst you talk about these things as if you're writing your grocery shopping list. I'm not saying that the person who did it was impersonal; she was lovely. She cares and understood how distressing this all is. It's just a lot to cope with. But if you're in Australia and in a similar position to me, I recommend you do it, if not for you for your loved ones. It's frigging scary saying these things out loud and then writing it down and signing it.

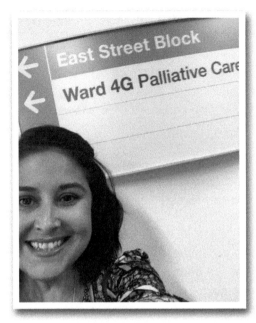

28 May 2016
Lisa in the Palliative Care ward
at Ipswich Hospital, QLD.

You see, I confront the fact that I am dying every day. People talk about it and I joke about it. That's all bravado. It's me not really accepting it. I'd rather joke about it than cry about it. But I definitely don't want to have to answer those detailed stupid questions again. So I'm hoping it was third time lucky and I never have to see my AHD EVER AGAIIN!!!!

Today was nice, and tomorrow will be easier. The fact that I just said tomorrow speaks volumes as two weeks ago I didn't think I would have a tomorrow.

Lisa coming home from hospital was always met with mixed emotions. Without a doubt we wanted her home as we knew this was her preference. But at this stage of the disease, we also worried that she was home a little too soon. Lisa got extremely good at convincing the palliative care team that she was feeling a lot better. Once her pain levels were under control (as under control as they could be) and her bowels had moved the slightest bit, she was packing to come home. This could be frightening at times. As much as I knew she would be a little temperamental when she got home, the first couple of days were always challenging. I remember reading this blog for the first time and having a lightbulb moment. Up until now I couldn't understand how someone who fought so hard to get home was always miserable for the first couple of days of getting home. Now it made sense.

Part of Lisa's issue was lack of patience. As soon as she would walk in the front door, she'd want to be up and about. She wanted to be normal. At the back of her mind she knew she had to recuperate but she resisted resting. Unfortunately for her, what she wanted to do and what she was fit to do were two different things. She would soon end up back in bed with increased pain medication and that feeling of despair. I couldn't help but feel sorry for her and wished to God we could swap places.

On top of adjusting to being back home, we were once again faced with updating the health care directive. On this occasion, I was so glad the social worker was there and went into a lot of detail to ensure we knew the repercussions of each decision. As Lisa previously stated, it's not like it is portrayed on television. Performing CPR on a body riddled with cancer would not be pretty. The likelihood was it would do more damage than good. These were the details we needed to hear and understand if we were to make informed decisions.

Somehow that day changed both our perceptions of what steps should be taken should Lisa be nearing the end of life. As hard as it was, I was relieved that the actions agreed to were clear. I would not be put in the position of having to decide whether Lisa would live or die. Lisa had made those decisions already and I was truly thankful.

> I would not be put in the position of having to decide whether Lisa would live or die.

Struggle Street Week

30/05/2016

So I've been struggling over the last few days with cognitive impairment and hand-eye coordination. My brain is basically like mush, and the ability to write anything, even a shopping list, has eluded me. It's been breaking my heart as my blogging is really what's been getting me through the last few weeks. So the thought of not being able to do it has been killing my life!!!!!

I woke up at 5am to yet another drug-induced nightmare. This time it was a girl with long black hair and a long white nighty that covered her feet, crawling towards the TV. I luckily fought my way out of that dream. You know that feeling? With a little bit of a yelp, I woke myself up, rolled over and picked up my phone. I scrolled through my *Terminally Fabulous* Facebook messages and one stood out.

It was from a young woman, Jess, also with a similar type of cancer to me. Jess is 24 and she says she's determined to make a quarter century. I say, why stop there? Be selfish, go for the century. Sir Donald Bradman wouldn't have stopped at 25! (Please note: I know this beautiful lady is striving for higher than that, but sometimes we need to set small goals to get to the big goals.) This beautiful young woman proceeded to discuss her symptoms in her comments. I had to keep stopping and typing to her that I had the exact same. Then I'd read another sentence, stop, message her that I too was the same, and this went on and on.

Jess is currently in another country, trying a last-ditch attempt at, I would presume, a cure, not just pain management or a short remission. I say more power to her. People have suggested these things to me over the years, but I'm just not one of those people who will start a six-week kiwi fruit cleanse whilst bathing in manuka honey and chanting chakras to an open fire. It's just not me. So far, my choices have been the right ones for me other than the immunotherapy. That stuff gave me high hopes at a high cost, and sadly it caused me more harm than good. But that is the risk you take with these things. You're damned if you do and you're damned if you don't!

Receiving Jess's message this morning has given me a renewed vigour. Our similarities (cancer symptoms wise) are uncanny, and I can just feel her energy through her message. She's like me, not a lie down. A just-take-it kinda girl and I love that! Good luck, my beautiful warrior, and I will see you when you get back to Oz.

Speaking of unexpected relationships. As a result of this 'shituation', through Instagram I've connected with another young woman named Roni, who's in her twenties with stage 4 cancer. She is a vivacious and talented photographer who has this amazing smile that would light up any dark day. She has been fighting for quite some time. We've been messaging back and forth for months now, and just the other day we bit the bullet and talked face to face via the wonderful world of Facebook video chat. Words cannot begin to describe the spirit and warmth that exudes from this young woman. We spoke nonstop, or maybe I did ... I don't know. All I know is there were no awkward moments of silence; it just flowed naturally.

One thought that is always at the back of my mind is: What about when I die? Who will keep me company for another 40 years before my mum or dad join me in Club Heaven? (no crocs allowed in my club heaven, by the way) Especially in the past week, that thought has been weighing heavily on my mind, and I have been struggling terribly.

I know not all of you will believe that there's a big party in the sky waiting for us, and to be quite honest, I'm not 100 per cent sure of it myself. But it gives me some comfort knowing that while you guys are left down here toiling away at work and stressing at everyday stresses, I'm up there with a bunch of family and old friends sipping ... who am I kidding ... SCULLING from a bottle of really expensive champagne, playing charades with Robin Williams, Audrey Hepburn and Patrick Swayze (yes Johnny!) and eating never-ending amounts of gluten. (Here on earth I'm coeliac. In heaven you can eat whatever you want, whenever you want!) And that's what usually gets me through. But not this week. Until I spoke with Roni, that is.

This is going to sound morbid, but the thought of someone like Roni maybe joining me up there gave me some comfort and peace of mind. Now don't get me wrong, I'm not wishing the end of this amazing woman's life, just so I can have a BFF up in the sky. Far from it. I wish for her, like I do every cancer sufferer, a cure. It just gave me comfort, and that was all I needed at that point in time.

This week has been an emotional rollercoaster to say the least, and I'm still on it. I've had immense highs: Constance Hall and her bestie Annaliese were part of my surprise blind date that Mum was in on organising. Obviously, this is at the top of that list of highs. I have been blessed with meeting or talking with four completely different women in total (Con, Annaliese, Jess and Roni). Each of them has brought something different to the table, but they all have one thing in common. They are strong warriors who don't take shit from anyone. Every time they get knocked down, they get up again. And if that isn't special, I don't know what is.

So to you, Con, Annaliese, Roni and Jess, I thank you. I thank you for having the courage to reach out to a complete stranger and share your most intimate stories with me. We now have a bond that no-one else could ever understand. In this world of cancer uncertainty, it's nice to know I now have four Fabulous Rockstars in my life to turn to.

What have I taken from this week?

> Be open to new possibilities because they could quite literally change your life.

Be open to new possibilities because they could quite literally change your life. I know my life has changed this week, and definitely for the better, even if my head is still mush, my vision blurred and my bowels slow. I'm in a better place today than I was last week. Maybe next week I will be in an even better place again.

Today I go in for a bout of radiation, and I go in with my head held high in the hope that maybe, just maybe, it's my turn for that miracle.

It took me quite a while to understand how quickly Lisa formed relationships with people that two days ago she didn't know existed. I never questioned them, but I had doubts about how real they were and how long they'd last. Lisa had lost so much to cancer; the last thing I wanted was for her to lose people she considered friends.

I had known of Constance Hall through her blog. I knew she had over a million followers and was extremely popular with young mums facing the everyday challenges of motherhood. From what I knew of her I could see a little of Lisa in Constance's writing. They were both honest beyond belief, not thinking twice about publicly writing what others probably thought but would never say out loud. I remember how shocked Lisa was when Con first contacted her about her blog. Lisa was not one to cling to someone for their popularity or accomplishments, but she absolutely loved how Con had made a success from what started out like any other blog, especially considering her honest approach and ability to swear like a trooper – a trait Lisa had also adopted when writing.

Unlike anyone else, Con was able to build Lisa's confidence about her writing, and she was so taken by it she shared Lisa's blog. The impact of this was amazing, Lisa's followers (Rockstars, as Lisa liked to refer to them) increased and the feedback was incredible. Lisa was so grateful to Con for her support and they became close online friends.

One day I received a private message from Con, asking me to help her arrange a surprise meeting with Lisa and Con's best friend Annaliese. Anyone that knows Lisa will know that Lisa does not deal well with surprises. I started laying the seed with Lisa by creating reasons to go into the city the following weekend. I was hit with a barrage of reasons why this was too difficult. It wasn't going to be easy.

One thing you learn from living with cancer is that irrespective of the lengths you go to plan anything, there are no guarantees. On the morning of Con's visit, Lisa was in extreme pain. When the palliative nurse called, Lisa was already dressed and ready to go to the city. Although she was originally resistant, pain or no pain, she was determined to go and do some shopping. After much negotiation with the palliative nurse, it was agreed that she could go but must be in the hospital by 5pm. Given that Constance had flown in from Perth and Annaliese from Sydney, you can imagine the relief I felt when this was agreed. I also knew that once Lisa found out that they had come all this way to visit her, she'd have been heartbroken if it hadn't been possible.

As soon as the girls met, I began to understand the power of online friendships. It was like meeting long-lost friends; the love and concern they had for Lisa was overwhelming. You see, once cancer invites itself into your home, life becomes extremely lonely. You, the cancer patient, lose the ability to come and go as you please, and life revolves around appointments, medication and unexpected visits to the emergency department. But there's more to it than that. Friends and family still have work to go to, lives to lead and families to care for. Without a doubt you remain a priority, but the reality is you are not their only priority. And when they do make time to visit, given Lisa is up to it physically and mentally, if it has been a tough week it's hard to bounce back and perk up for visitors.

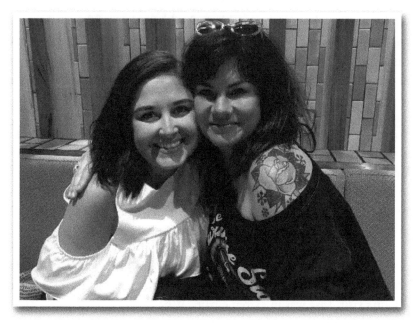

19 September 2016
Lisa catching up with Constance Hall at Perth Airport, WA.

We had been on the terminal journey for two years at this stage. It felt like one constant balancing act, keeping friends close whilst being able to hide away from the world when you just weren't up for it. For the girls to have flown to Brisbane just to spend two hours with Lisa was priceless. They knew there was a risk that they may not even see Lisa on that day, considering how her health had been for the past three months. But they took the risk.

Lisa was absolutely blown away by it all, as was I. From that day forward, they both became an important part of our close circle of friends. They were always a message or a call away, to listen on our toughest days and to laugh with on our best days. I'm so glad our friendship has continued since Lisa's passing.

As for Roni, this beautiful girl remained close friends with Lisa throughout her cancer journey. Who else better to discuss the highs and lows of this ugly disease than someone who fully understands what you are going through? Roni, I'm also pleased to say, is NED (No Evidence of Disease) at the moment. She is living life to the full and enjoying every single minute of it.

Sadly, Jess passed away on 4th July 2016. I have no doubt in my mind that Jess and Lisa will be up above, sipping that expensive champagne Lisa talks about and laughing at her mum trying to write a book. Strange as it seems, it gives me comfort knowing the girls have each other.

Men Have Feelings Too: Well, at Least I Think They Do

07/06/2016

How are you going?

How's your mum going?
How does Ava cope with it all? Does she understand what's going on?
How does Marianne take it?
How's your nan?
How is your aunty taking it?
How is Rebecca coping?

I don't know if you've noticed the common element here. When it comes to being asked questions about how people are affected by my cancer, they tend to be directed towards the women in my life. I believe there is a reason for this.

I think it is because it tends to be women that actually ask how people around me are being affected by the cancer. This doesn't only apply to cancer; women ask questions about EVERYTHING.

Men are simple creatures, really. If a man is on the phone, when he completes his call you can ask him how the person on the other end of the phone was. What are they up to? What were you talking about? How are their family? Where have they been lately? How's work going for them? Did they end up going with the floating floor boards or tiles? The general response will be firstly a look that says, "What the fuck are you talking about, woman? It's not the bloody Spanish Inquisition". This will be followed by "I don't know. We don't talk about that shit," and usually a shrug of the shoulders.

What, you don't talk about life?

Our response as naturally caring, nosy bitches is usually, "What do you mean you don't know? You've just been on the phone to him for 30 minutes and you don't even know if he got over the flu yet or how he's feeling... huh? What do you guys actually talk about? You couldn't have spent the last half an hour talking about last week's game and how the ref was obviously the other team's supporter blah blah fuckity blah. I told you when you took the call that your mission was to confirm or deny the rumour that I heard at Pilates this morning from Susie's friend Claire, who knows Mary, who knows Tina, who works at your mate's office at reception, who said she overheard your mate talking to divorce lawyers the other day in his office about divorcing Sarah." (Note: Sarah is the made-up wife of the made-up husband of my made-up boyfriend's mate, and this whole scenario is made up for dramatic effect.)

As good gossipers, we as women always have stories to tell the men in our lives after a convo with our girlfriend. Yes, even when we swear on our friendship that we won't tell a soul, we always at least tell one. Come on, we all do it. You guys just don't admit to it. We can't help it. We are natural 'storytellers' – not gossipers just relaters of stories. And as good story-sharing bitches, just once we'd like a little bit of return gossip game from the men in our lives. Is that too much to ask? I know you've all been there at one point in your lives, looking at your guy, thinking, *How the fuck do you people manage to function in day-to-day life if you don't even fucking know if your friend is doing alright?*

So this I believe is one of the reasons the men in my life seemingly go unnoticed when it comes to people asking how they're affected by my illness. The most obvious reason is their usual inability to emote. Men are meant to be the protectors, the ones who don't cry, the ones who bravely run out in their undies at 11pm to eradicate a cockroach, even though they're shit-scared of them. They're the ones who get up to check that imaginary bump in the night we heard. They are our big, brave protectors, not mushy, emotional talk-about-their-feelings wimps. Or do we not give them enough credit? Just because they're not running around practising their crying face in the mirror like us doesn't mean they don't go into the shower and have a secret man-cry.

I for one can only speak about the two closest men in my life — my father and my brother.

My brother Steven is what I would call a 'thinker', a 'fixer'. His natural response is to google, investigate and look for answers, and that's how he deals with things. (This is purely my opinion; he may think completely differently.) We've discussed it to a point, the cancer, I mean. There are days that I will just force it down his throat, and to his credit he listens and usually retorts with some sort of uplifting fact or quote — because that's what he does. He 'fixes'.

I can't remember seeing him cry. I'm sure he has. I'm sure he does. You see, my brother and I, like any family, are genetically placed together, and of course we love each other. I know I would crawl over broken glass for him. I would die for him. I've always loved him. I was obsessed with him as a kid. I loved holding his hand and used to sneak into his bed at night when I was shit-scared of the dark. Our personalities are completely different, and there are days we could kill each other and days we are the best people in each other's lives. So I would say we have a perfectly normal, functioning brother-sister relationship.

So if someone was to ask how my brother is, I would respond, "All bravado with a side of shit-scared". I know he hates that I'm going through this. I know it breaks his heart. He's just like most men and internalises his pain and fear. So for those who want to know, that is my answer. Like the rest of us he is scared; he just may not quite know it yet.

Now when it comes to my dad, well, that breaks my heart! To say he is heartbroken is the biggest understatement of the year. My dad has continued to work throughout my whole cancer treatment. Work is my dad's way of coping. It's his way of escaping the reality that is our life of cancer.

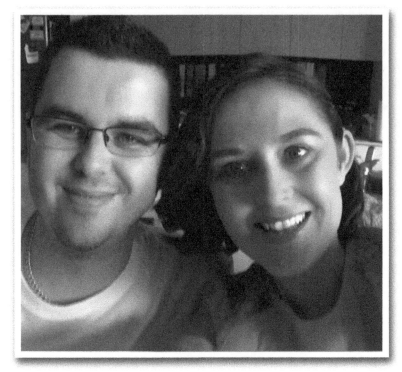

Christmas Day 2015
Lisa and Steven at home in Springfield Lakes, QLD.

When we were kids, Mum's work hours were never ending, but Dad had shift work. So more often than not he would be the one who was home first, and at the weekends he was the one that shaved my legs for the first time while Mum was at work. He was the one that told me about periods and pads while Mum was at work. He was the one I would tell my secrets to. But sadly I allowed outside forces to break down our once ironclad relationship.

You see, he and my former partner didn't get on, but he never once stopped loving me throughout that whole ordeal. I'm sure, though, there were many a tear cried even pre-cancer because of our broken relationship. When it came to my illness over the last four years, Dad has been treated like a second-class citizen because of the dynamic with my ex (not because of myself, my mum, my family or friends). He was basically made to feel like a stranger in his own daughter's life. He was made to feel uncomfortable by my hospital bedside. When he would visit me, it was like he was on the outside looking in, and he wasn't allowed in the front door. For him this would have been heart-breaking as we always had an incredibly close, loving, honest and caring relationship.

So how is my dad doing?

He is broken. He breaks down at the sight of me in pain, which is often. If he accompanies me to the hospital, he will always cry. He would do anything for me and he does. Our relationship? Well, thankfully, since moving back home it is as it was before – a strong, loving relationship with a mutual respect and admiration for one another, which I believe is like no other. Don't get me wrong; we still drive each other up the wall with both our stubborn I-always-have-to-be-right attitude. And I don't know how one human being can make so much noise. He's constantly rattling and tapping. But we love each other, and sadly he knows that one day he won't be able to 'annoy' me anymore, like he so loves to do.

Just remember: Men have feelings too. They're just not bright enough to realise it.

> Men have feelings too. They're just not bright enough to realise it.

One thing was for sure, we all dealt with Lisa's cancer differently. Looking back it's hard to say exactly how we each dealt with it as cancer is an ever-moving target. When the news was good, obviously we were ecstatic. But unfortunately those times were few and far between.

Steven and Lisa were extremely close in many ways, but their arguing at times was relentless, even in the later stages of Lisa's illness. This concerned me greatly as I always worried that Lisa would pass, and Steven would be left feeling regret and guilt. I mentioned this to Steven many times, but he found it increasingly difficult to cope with Lisa's communication at times. When in pain she became demanding and really struggled to control her frustrations. This was completely understandable, but Steven found it difficult to accept this and would often verbalise his annoyance. This made life extremely difficult for me as I always felt like the meat in the sandwich.

I could understand Steven's annoyance, but having lived with Lisa, watched her suffering and diminishing quality of life 24/7, I came to accept that there had to be a way for her to relieve her frustrations. Through time I'd developed extremely high tolerance levels. I'm not saying there were no tears and hurt – there were plenty – but mainly in the privacy of my own room.

On the flip side, when Lisa was in hospital and the news was not good, Steven was just like the rest of us. Worry and despair weighed heavily on him. Lisa is right; his way of coping was to google for answers. Unbeknown to Lisa, though, Steven wasn't always looking for a magic treatment or a new trial. By this stage in Lisa's disease we all knew these were no longer options. Steven was googling to see what Lisa's symptoms were telling us, what stage of the cancer journey she was at, if it was safe to go to work tomorrow, and to know whether Lisa would still be with us when he returned to the hospital after work.

I made my own conclusions by what the doctor was telling us, and I often said to Steven that I didn't think Lisa would make it out of the hospital this time. But Steven remained optimistic as Google had reassured him that Lisa would once again turn a corner and be home in a day or two. Thankfully, the majority of times Google was right.

Peter was different to us all and found it impossible to put on a macho front. Lisa's closeness with her dad had been restored after her break-up with her ex. I knew that Lisa loved me and that when she was really hurting, I was the one she needed. But her dad was the one she confided in. Growing up she would tell him what was going on in her life, so he could break it to me gently as I was the worrier, the stressed one. I thought situations through and worried about the longer-term impact; Peter lived for the day. Dealing with Lisa's prognosis was no different. Peter in some ways refused to accept what we knew was in front of us. He couldn't discuss what lay ahead, and when I tried to have these talks, he would fall apart and politely refuse to go there.

Many times, in the emergency department when Lisa was crying out in pain, I would pray to God to end her pain in whatever way possible. I just couldn't bear the thought of her continuously going through this excruciating agony. But while Peter didn't want her to suffer, he wasn't prepared to lose her either.

It's Not the Natural Order of Things

14/06/2016

Man meets woman, or in my parent's case, teenage boy throws one metre by one metre advertising sandwich board at teenage girl's head whom he finds attractive, believing this to be some sort of natural mating call.

So, let's just say, it was not love at first sight. It took another meeting for Mum and Dad to actually start the dating ritual. Mum and Dad were 16 and 17 at the time, and both very inexperienced. They'd both had boyfriends and girlfriends, I'm sure, but we're talking kissing behind the bike sheds at school type relationships. The good old kiss and dump – nothing serious. Like, if it was 2016, neither of them would have ever updated their status to 'In a relationship'.

So Boy and Girl (Peter and Geraldine) quickly become inseparable. They both go to different schools and live in different little country towns in Ireland, but they make it work. Then it happens. Boy and Girl find out they're having a little boy or girl themselves.

Poor Geraldine, she must have been petrified. She was on holiday in Canada at the time, visiting family, and she was constantly feeling ill. One day at the kitchen sink, Geraldine's mum turns to Geraldine and asks probably every parent's worst nightmare of their 16-year-old daughter: "Is there a chance you could be pregnant?" Now what you also have to remember is this was the 1980s and my Mum was being brought up in a strict Irish Catholic family. Catholic school, Mass every Sunday, weekly confessions – everything from leaving your teabag in the pot too long to leaving the toilet seat up is a mortal sin. We Irish Catholics do love ourselves a bit of good old religious guilt. The fear of God is instilled in us from no age, and the fear of your father ... well, second to the fear of God. "Wait until your father hears this" must be six of the scariest words known to any child, let alone a now 16-year-old who thinks she is pregnant.

Geraldine's mother insists on marching her down to a local pharmacy to purchase a pregnancy test. Lo and behold, Geraldine is pregnant. Hello future *Terminally Fabulous* Lisa Magill.

My future mum and dad do the right thing and get married. Mum wears a gorgeous lace curtain design and her sister and cousin wear a just as fabulous lacy blush pink floor-length, neck-high dress that would make a Sister Wife look like a tart. I'm front row at the wedding (literally, as I was in Mum's belly and had a belly button view). A few months later, along comes moi. Second to probably the chocolate Galaxy Ripple, I like to think I was the best thing to ever happen to my mum at that point in her life.

Mum and Dad took to marriage like ducks to water. Sure they struggled. They lived in Department of Housing. Dad got a fitter machinist apprenticeship and Mum worked in the afternoons as a cleaner at a hospital for the physically and mentally disabled. I never went hungry, I never went naked, and most importantly, I never went unloved.

My parents could have chosen any number of options when they found out they were pregnant with me, and we obviously don't need to go into them. But they didn't. They chose to get permission to marry under age and then move out of home straight away to raise me. They took on the complete responsibility from the first moment that little pink positive sign rocked up. For that I will be forever grateful and proud of my parents. They will be celebrating their 35th wedding anniversary on the 9th of July this year, and yes, I do like to take credit for being the best matchmaker in the world. If it weren't for me, these two lovebirds may never have lasted ... You can thank me later, Mum and Dad.

So we fast forward some 30 odd years and I make the phone call to Mum advising her that my cancer is back and I'm effectively dying: WRONG ORDER!!!!!!

This is not how it is meant to work. Mum and Dad look after their children until adulthood (well, they never really stop at all), and your grandparents start to get greyer, a little slower and start to replace joints in their body. The younger ones look after the older ones, not the other way around.

A couple of weeks ago, when we had what feels like our hundredth scare in palliative care, my poor grandmother, along with my aunty, rushed to my bedside from Ireland. I've now been told on three separate occasions in hospital that I will not be walking out and will most likely be pushed out on a bed, feet first with a discreet sheet pulled over my head. Well, that's how I imagined it, but apparently you are placed in a secret hidey hole underneath what looks like a bed. So you wouldn't even know there is a dead body being concealed.

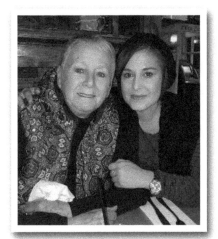
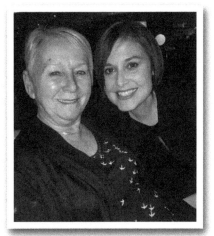
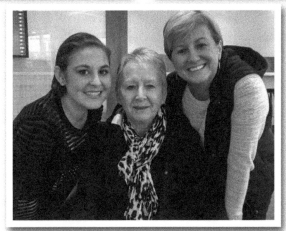

Unbeknownst to the family, Lisa planned a trip to Tasmania when her Gran was here on holiday. Another beautiful trip ticked off her bucket list.

My grandmother is not the bubbly, vivacious woman with a wickedly dirty sense of humour that she once was. She once told me not to spend all my birthday money on porn, to which I informed her that you can get all that stuff for free now on the internet. Her response: "So where does one get this internet thing then?" Sadly, old age has started to take her away from me. I don't think she fully understands the gravity of my current situation. In some way, I am grateful for this because I just don't believe she could handle it. For as long as I have known her, my gran has always been joking.

"You'll regret speaking to your grandmother like this when I'm pushing up the daisies!" Well, here we are again: WRONG ORDER!!!!! There are occasions where my gran will have moments of clarity and break down about what's happening to me, and it's just not right. It's not how things are meant to go, and this breaks her heart. This bitch of a cancer is making my gran cry and that pisses me off.

My poor grandad, like my brother, is a fixer. He still uses a thing called 'teletext' (a thing on the TV similar to internet that gives news updates, the weather and the like), and occasionally there will be some sort of cancer cure update. So he'll rush to the phone and tell me of this new miracle. Sadly, my grandad cannot travel due to a heart problem, and I know this also breaks his heart that he cannot be by my side. That's all he really wants, to hug his granddaughter and make it all better. Again, WRONG ORDER!!!!!

The biggest WRONG ORDER, though, is that of parents facing the thought of burying their own child. WRONG ORDER!!!!!!

My parents were meant to age gracefully and get to a stage where I would have built a granny flat or have a house big enough for us all to live in. I would then proceed to wipe my mum's bum, like she did for me when I was a baby. Mum is not meant to be putting suppositories up her 34-year-old daughter's butt.

My mum and dad are not meant to be discussing eulogies and possible burial sites for their daughter. My parents are not meant to be waking in the middle of the night to go and listen at their daughter's bedroom door, to check if she is still breathing. These are the things I was meant to be doing for my parents in 25 years' time, not the other way around.

My Mum and Dad will eventually only have one child. When people ask them that question, "So how many kids do you have?" what will they answer? ... "Well, we did have two, but cancer took one away"...?

Cancer doesn't give a shit about natural order. Why should any parent lose their child? There is no rhyme or reason as to how all this shit works, other than to say it's just the WRONG ORDER!

> Cancer doesn't give a shit about natural order.

Stay Fabulous, Rockstars.

And for all of you fabulous people out there, I hope you never have to use the words 'IT'S JUST THE WRONG ORDER!'

One thing we knew for sure when Lisa started the blog was that nothing would remain private. But if I'm being honest, nothing in our house remained a secret for too long. Somehow the kids knew from an early age that I was 16 and pregnant when Peter and I got married. However, I don't think we ever discussed with them just how difficult that was for both of us.

Although going it alone wasn't easy, once we'd emigrated to Australia we settled well and always knew we had made the right decision for our family. We loved our new way of life and worked hard to achieve the great Aussie dream. We were happy. Fast forward 35 years, and we thought the tougher times of bringing up a family were behind us. We now knew what truly hard times were. Our daughter was dying and all the hard work in the world wouldn't change this.

We had always missed our family and friends, but in all honesty, we had made many wonderful friends. So distance never seemed like such a big deal until now. We felt lonely and isolated, with no mum and dad popping in to see how we were coping. No sisters or brothers were living close by to offer a helping hand. Our ability to go it alone was truly challenged, and at times we struggled mentally and physically. I know I've mentioned it before but thank God for true friends. They were, and still are, our lifeline.

Without a doubt, the first thing to come to mind when Lisa was diagnosed as terminal was why her and why not me. And I know Peter felt the same. As anyone will tell you that has lost or is losing a child (irrespective of their age), it is definitely one of the hardest things you will ever have to go through. The cruelty of having to watch them deteriorate before your very eyes is soul-destroying. I remember walking through the shopping centre many times and feeling jealous of what looked like happy families, laughing and seemingly having fun whilst I was on a mercy dash to pick up some prescriptions. If I passed someone in a headscarf, looking pasty with no eyebrows, I wanted to run over, give them a hug and tell them I knew exactly what they were going through. Just so they would know they weren't on their own.

Nothing in life prepares you for this. As hard as it was for us, I knew it was just as hard for our family back home. I can only imagine how they must have felt being so far away and not knowing what was going on from one day to the next. The difficulty for us was in deciding when they should be contacted. If we'd contacted them with every scare, they'd have spent their time coming back and forth to Australia at least every month. I remember praying hard at night that no other family would be going through what we were going through, but sadly I knew that wasn't the case.

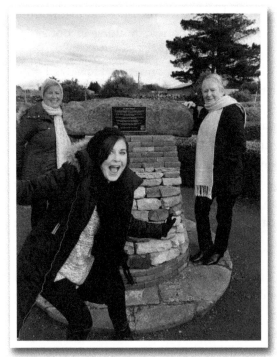

28 July 2015
Geraldine, Lisa and her granny Ellen during
a family sightseeing trip in Tasmania.

Give Us All Your Money or Die

18/06/2016

So, I have been tossing up whether to post this for a while now. It's not to be controversial or to lambast the drug companies that provide so many people with lifesaving or life-extending drugs. But I just feel the need to get this out there. This is all, of course, 'speculation' and just my opinion.

Drug companies have no problem taking our hard-earned money – most of us who are in terminal cancer stages specifically. They certainly have us by the short and curlies. (Note: for those of you born post 2000, this is slang for pubic hair. Again, this is hair that grows on your nether regions to help protect you from bacterial infections, also known as the map of Tasmania, bush, landing strip, carpet etc.) Obviously, this happens with other illnesses such as MS, Parkinson's and ulcerated colitis. People need these drugs to survive and the drug companies know it.

For those of us who have ran out of traditional treatment options, we mortgage our houses, sell our children's kidney (joke!), secretly post our husband's prized signed Muhammad Ali fight gloves on Gumtree to try and raise funds for treatment, or we set up GoFundMe campaigns, which for many is embarrassing and demeaning. Asking for money is hard. Sadly, for those that need it most, often their pride gets in the way and they'd rather live on baked beans than ask a friend, let alone a stranger for financial help.

Basically, it's a treat-or-die situation, and if you're told there is a drug that has shown really good promise for your cancer, or something similar to the genetic makeup of your cancer, of course you'd sell your soul to the devil to try this new 'miracle' drug. Sadly, these drugs are quite often not the panacea we are promised they will be. But we as cancer patients jump on them because they offer us that word again: hope. It's the one thing that we clutch onto with our fingernails whilst we sit in chemo chairs for hours on end having toxic sludge pumped into our veins, holding onto sick bags, with our heads aching and cold from losing our hair to this miracle drug.

> Hope. It's the one thing that we clutch onto with our fingernails.

Our bodies are either bloated or emaciated, and all because a doctor has advised us this could be the lifesaving drug we have been waiting for.

Don't get me wrong. I am grateful for these new treatment options, and I for one am one of those people who jumps on most treatment options offered. They are offered to me few and far between for my never-before-seen cancer. So as you can imagine, the drug companies don't spend much money on trying to find a cure for just one person. It just doesn't make sense economically or time wise when they could be putting their energies, and most importantly money, into something that could save thousands.

Immunotherapy seems to be the next big thing in cancer treatment, and here is my concern. One drug that I was offered cost around $7000 every three weeks. If you were eligible the drug company would pay every second treatment for a total of three each. They tend to treat you with six of these intravenous treatments over 18 weeks and then scan you to see if there is improvement.

Now this drug, like all drugs, has a myriad of side effects that can occur. One was that it can make your tumours grow before it shrinks them. The only problem was they may grow but not shrink back to what they were, or smaller. It can also cause permanent lung damage as immunotherapy can start to attack the healthy tissue of your organs, which is what happened to me. We stopped after three treatments as the risks outgrew the possible reward of the drug in my case.

Herein lies my problem: I was told to try this drug because I had a good reaction to radiation, which is very rare for a person at my point of disease. So we worked out the costs. I was in a health fund at the time and, thankfully, they paid half of my fee for each treatment that I had to pay for. The thing is, now I'm seeing this treatment offered EVERYWHERE. So many people who read this blog write to me about it and the cost involved and the funding they need to get it and so on. But when I ask them why this drug was suggested to be beneficial for them, they don't know.

This drug has thrown melanoma treatment on its head and has it in a choke hold for the first time ever. It actually puts people in remission that were given no hope, where the disease had spread to their bones and vital organs. In previous times this basically meant you're fucked, but this drug has shown so much promise.

But did you know that the drug companies that make these drugs wine and dine specialists in order to get their new drug out there? Did you know specialists are attending conferences in places like Vienna and Vancouver and the list goes on?

According to the Sydney Morning Herald, one company spent $285,732 sending 24 oncologists to a five-day conference in Chicago with more than $10,000 spent on dinner allowance. Here's a link to the article, if you're interested http://m.smh.com.au/national/health/pharmaceutical-companies-splash-43-million-on-health-professionals-in-six-months-20160329-gnsy45.html, which has much more interesting and expensive reading.

My whole point is to show you the power of the almighty dollar over life. Very few people can afford $7000 every three weeks for a drug that holds no guarantee for them. And then what if it does work? Oh, happy days. But how is the average Joe going to be able to afford to pay these exorbitant fees for an unknown period of time? What if this drug keeps them going until they're 85? Not everyone is James Packer with an endless money supply.

Money should not determine life, and the fact that the deciding factor for many drug companies to proceed with making certain drugs is whether they will make money is disgusting to me. I'd like to see a big drug company CEO sitting by the bedside of their bald, violently ill, dying 34-year-old daughter who is in 24/7 pain and simply deny them the chance at life because their disease isn't common enough, so the costs of making the drug outweigh the return of selling it. And to those specialists that have been practising the you-scratch-my-back-and-I'll-scratch-yours since the dawn of time, maybe next time when you're sipping on your cocktail in Puerto Rico, while your patient is back home scrimping the money together to pay for this new miracle treatment, you might think twice about pushing the new drug on your patient just 'because'.

Remember, this is life or death for us, not "Should I go for the Pina Colada or the Espresso Martini?"

I also want to let you know that this, like many things, does not apply to every oncologist or drug company. This is just something that has been brought up more and more by you fabulous readers, and it breaks my heart knowing that some of you will die because a drug is not on the PBS and you simply can't afford it.

> Life over dollar, not dollar over life. It should be humanity over monetary.

Life over dollar, not dollar over life. It should be humanity over monetary. Just think of how many people may have died while you were reading this because they can't afford treatment. Doesn't feel right, does it?

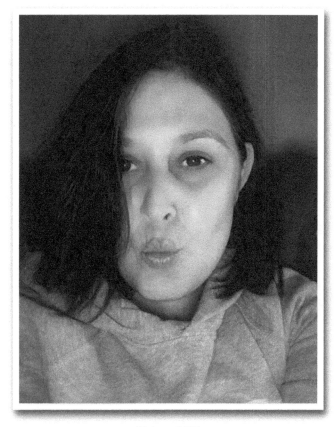

17 June 2016
Another milestone reached... moving into our new house. We never thought Lisa would be around to see it being built let alone move in.

The Longest Blog About Nothing

22/06/2016

The Longest Blog About Nothing in the History of the Longest Blogs About Nothing (Seinfeld Would be Proud)

I don't want to die with people hating me. These are words I never thought would cross my mind and never mind leave my mouth. But it was triggered by something my friend said the other day to me, and it cut. It cut deep, probably because I had already been thinking it myself. She said if I died tomorrow, she'd rather I died the way our relationship was and how I was six months ago, not how I am now. I totally understand where she's coming from. She didn't just blurt it out of nowhere. We were actually addressing our newly challenged/changed relationship in an environment where these sorts of issues are meant to be addressed.

Cancer brings a lot more than just pain, tumours and hair loss. It affects every relationship you're involved in, with your mother, father, brother, sister, in-laws, cousins, friends, workmates and even your local newsagent. It has a way of working its way into your life like haemorrhoids. You don't know where they come from. They just pop up one day and start to be a real pain in the arse. Let's just say if there was a Facebook friendship relationship status update, my friend who made the comment and I would be currently under 'It's complicated but we're working on it'. This bastard of a thing will not wreck my relationship with this person. My love and admiration for them is too deep for this cancer to ever fuck it up. So up yours, cancer; your little plan isn't working.

I get it; I totally do. These drugs I am on, if you were taking them individually, your emotions would be all over the place like a North Queensland summer's day. You wake up in the morning at 7am all sunny and singing. By 11am it's overcast and raining. At 1pm you're out frolicking and having fun at the beach. Then it hits 5pm again and the thunder starts to roll in, the lightning starts to strike and the rain begins to set in. Finally, by 9pm you're relaxing on the balcony watching the moon shine between the clouds and listening to the calming sounds of the ocean. Then, just like your iPhone music, you hit repeat and shuffle the next day and it starts all over again. You see, I never know which Lisa I am going to get at any given time of the day, and my friends certainly don't either. As you can imagine this would put some strain on any relationship.

I like to think I've always been a pretty decent person, the type of person who, at the cash register, lets the person with five items go in front of me, even if I only have like 12. I prefer to give than receive. I used to save my birthday and Christmas money for presents for other people's birthdays and special occasions when I was younger. I'm the type of person who will always wave thank you for letting me merge in traffic. I'm the one who always stands to the side in the shopping centre aisle Mexican stand-off, or that's who I was. Well, I sometimes still am.

I'm like a tsunami, completely unpredictable. I am more up and down emotionally than Oprah Winfrey's weight in the eighties. I have had more arguments in the last four months than Charlie Sheen has had porn stars and broken bed springs. The last thing I want is to die with my friends and family thinking, *Fuck, she was a bitch near the end there*. I want them to think, *Fuck, we've lost a good person. Fuck, I'm sad. Fuck, how will I live without her? Fire truck, I miss Lisa.* (That's Ava, my nearly three-year-old niece. She only swears when it's warranted or if she thinks no-one is listening.) *Fuck, how will I function as a fully functioning human being without Lisa in the world?* ... Okay, I may have gone a bit overboard there, but you get what I mean.

Throw in the 24-hour pain meds, nerve pain meds and other pain meds I am on, and the one to two hours' broken sleep I am lucky to get each night ...

I honestly don't know how people with chronic fatigue do it every day. How do they possibly force themselves out of bed feeling this way all the time? I have never felt tiredness like it. It is like I am walking in a cloud all day long. I have micro sleeps all day too. I'll just be sitting there and the next thing I am asleep. I have actually been in the midst of giving myself a needle and had a micro sleep, waking up with a syringe inches from my eye whilst attempting to administer my pain medication in the middle of the night.

I have no control at all over my thoughts or what comes out of my mouth or what I do. For example, I apparently phoned my friend Melissa the other day and asked her if she likes diamond earrings. Her response was

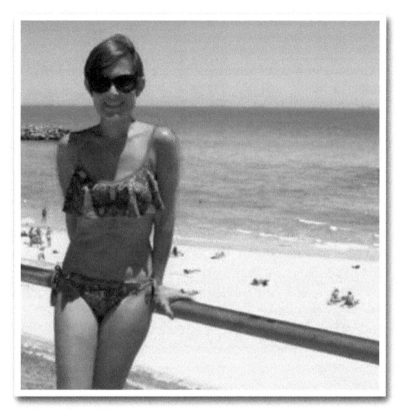

4 February 2015
Lisa always loved the beach.

"Yes of course, but why are you asking this?" to which I replied, "Things aren't looking good," and I simply hung up the phone. I have absolutely no recollection of this ever happening. I apparently also then rang my friend Rebecca and was discussing with her that her partner is a colorectal surgeon. The conversation ended quite quickly because Rebecca decided that I wasn't in my right mind and perhaps I needed to get off the phone to have a little bit of a sleep as I certainly wasn't making sense. And no, her partner is not a colorectal surgeon for the rectum, I mean record.

I've also been in the emergency department and asked the doctor in charge, who was probably only in is early thirties, how long he had been balding for. Was he balding since he was a young man? Mum says the ground could have swallowed her up. She said she feels like this on many an occasion, especially when I'm in hospital. I have also asked nurses and doctors to begin polygamist marriages with me in the emergency department.

So as you may have noticed, my thoughts are not always what you would call normal.

My mind, being as unpredictable as it is now, is also concerning me in relation to the future of my blog. I was only responding to a comment from a fellow blogger @youngmamadrama yesterday that the blogs that used to seemingly just pour from my brain through my fingertips onto my iPad, with general ease and enjoyment, are becoming more and more difficult to write. And this of course scares me. As you know, my blog is my outlet. It has become more to me than just an online diary. It has become a place where I can come to escape and relate to others in similar situations to myself. It has become more of a community – a support network for friends and a family of people who are going through hard times. Not necessarily cancer-related either. Maybe postnatal depression, maybe post-traumatic stress disorder, maybe just the daily stresses of life like motherhood and why your child won't eat a sandwich with the crust on today but yesterday she did. To lose the ability to communicate with you Fabulous Rockstars would just push me over the edge. It would totally break my heart.

I've already lost so much to this disease. I cannot work. I cannot just hop in the car to go grab that bottle of milk or to blast the music and sing loudly, just to escape my house for a minute. You know, when you need that break. I can't do that anymore. I could just go and sit in the car in the driveway and do it, but somehow, I don't think our new neighbours at our new house would appreciate some crazy psycho headbanging in the car next to their house. Although if they did it, I'd get some popcorn and enjoy the show!

So, like an episode of Seinfeld, this has been a blog about nothing really. Nothing bad or new has happened. Well, apart from my personality transplant and that we're now at a 14-kilo weight gain mark in just a few short months.

I haven't been told I have new tumours or that it has spread to the bones or the brain or the lungs. They're all still in the same place (as far as I'm aware of). I don't know exactly how many I have. We've sort of just stopped counting them now. I know there'd be at least 20 of the slippery suckers. I have this horrible fear that it will spread to one of those three areas. I don't care if it continues in the same way it has the last few years. Just stay the fuck away from my brain; I need that bastard to think. Stay away from my bones; my skin needs somewhere to hang around. And for fuck's sake, stay away from my lungs; I need those things to breathe.

I've had asthma all my life, but it was particularly bad as a child/teenager. I've been hospitalised with a quarter of my lungs working. I know what it's like to fight for every gasp of air you can get and not be able to go to sleep because you, firstly, can't lie down comfortably when you can't take a breath and, secondly, you're shit-scared you'll suffocate to death in the middle of the night. I don't want to be walking around with an oxygen tank on 24 hours a day, or worse still, being pushed around in a wheelchair with an oxygen tank!

Other than the fact that I feel I am no longer the nice, calm, dependable, giving, loving and caring person that I used to be, she's still there. She is just not there as often in a day as she used to be – more like six hours a day the old Lisa and eight hours a day the crankier Lisa. And the other ten hours, well, that's anybody's guess. I suppose the point of all this jibber jabber is to let those I love, and those I care about, those who've been around since day one and those of you whom I have only recently gotten to know through my blog, know that deep down I am still the same person I always was. You just have to dig a little bit deeper to find me now.

I promise I have realised these drugs I am taking alter my personality in a way that does not please me and others. So I am now working on it, as much as the drugs will allow me, to get the old Lisa back on track, if not for you for me. Because I miss knowing what mood I'm going to be in, and I miss the old bubbly, happy and sing-and-dance-in-the-shower Lisa. I promise she's still here and she will be back! I promise I'm not a total bitch. That sounded a bit like "Trust me, I'm a politician. Trust me, I have terminal cancer." All I can do is work on it.

> I miss the old bubbly, happy and sing-and-dance-in-the-shower Lisa.

The first step to fixing a problem is recognising there is one, and I've done that. So we're already on our way to Terminally Fabulous Lisa-land, and

I promise it will be better than Disneyland on steroids. (You see that? A little bit of steroid humour. Now I couldn't have joked about that when I started this blog. Now I'm making fun of the bastard, I'd say we're halfway to recovery already!)

Stay Fabulous, Rockstars.

When I think of the last ten years of Lisa's life, I see a change that started long before the cancer. I don't mean the short temper, the frustration and the anger, but I do believe Lisa started losing her bubbly, happy, outgoing personality that she was once known for. And as time went on, she found it harder and harder to be herself. Things were extremely difficult in her relationship and therefore her home life. She was isolated and at times extremely lonely. Socialising with friends was practically non-existent except for a rare catch-up over dinner. To top it off along came cancer with its relentless treatments and the cruel after-effects.

Although Peter and I struggled with both, the relationship problems and Lisa's diagnosis, as hard as it was, we never tried to tell her what to do. We let her live her life. One thing we had learnt about Lisa as we went through her teenage years was if we pushed one way, Lisa would push the other. And the last thing we needed or wanted was to subconsciously push Lisa away when she needed us most. As long as we stayed close, we knew she was safe.

The drug-induced changes in Lisa's temperament were unpredictable, but the reactions from these drugs also depended on the prescribed quantity and frequency. In some ways, I was prepared for the chain reaction. However, knowing what was about to go down and being able to cope with it are two very different things. Dexi was usually prescribed after a trip to emergency and a highly stressful 24 hours. So, as much as I knew things would become difficult after a day or two, I was also fragile and my ability to cope was extremely low.

I rarely reacted to Lisa's outbursts. To be perfectly frank, I don't think I had the energy as I was mentally drained. Unfortunately, this generally resulted in a lot of bottled-up emotions followed by tears. I had to remind myself on numerous occasions that it was cancer I was cross with for the constant cruelty it thrust upon Lisa, rather than Lisa herself. She had no control over what was happening, and it was eating her up inside. I could always tell how guilty Lisa felt after an outburst. I'd tell her often that when I'd look back on our time together, I'd only think of the good times. When her time was coming to an end, she needed to remind herself of this and I'd once again reiterate "No regrets".

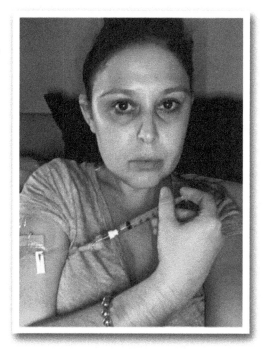

30 June 2016
Lisa at home having pain relief
in the middle of the night.

Now That You're Dying, What's Your Advice About Living?

04/07/2016

A question I am often asked is "What advice would you give to people who don't have cancer and how they should live their lives?"

This question always leaves me slightly speechless, because at the end of the day, no one person should ever be telling another person how they should live their life, whether they have terminal cancer or not. Just because I'm dying prematurely doesn't mean I have all the answers. Once you're diagnosed with a terminal disease, you don't get an email from God telling you the elusive answer to that elusive question: What does it all mean? What are we all really here for? It's as if once we are diagnosed, we become the go-to person for all things philosophical. Much to my own disappointment I don't hold the secret to life.

Don't get me wrong, I LOVE that people come to me for advice, and I'm always happy to give someone my two cents' worth. I just hope they understand I can only give my opinion, and that's not necessarily always right, or legal for that matter.

Of course, I always respond with the generic:

"Live every day as if it's your last."
"Don't sweat the small stuff."
"Hug your kids."
"Tell people you love them."
"Don't put off that trip to that place you've always wanted to go to."

.... the usual stuff. The stuff you already know, but you just don't always get around to doing it because, quite frankly, life and living get in the way.

These responses are the right ones. The things that we should be doing every day often get pushed aside for the dinging of a phone. It's that email that just can't wait until 9am tomorrow when you get into the office, just like that fax that used to wait in the tray for you until the next business day before email existed. Remember those days? The days before we didn't have a whole office set up in our pants. Our phones are exactly that: a portable office. I honestly wonder how kids get any attention from their parents and how parents get any attention from their kids these days.

Go into any household on any given night of the week and you will find an adult replying to an email on their Samsung Galaxy, another adult playing word games with friends on their iPhone, a kid feeding their virtual pet on their iPad and another kid upstairs with their headset on, communicating in some foreign techno language to a kid on the other side of the world on their Xbox. Now this I can honestly say is not living. It is not using life to its fullest potential. But we are all guilty of it. Put your hand up if you have been to a movie recently and been able to not look at your phone at least once during the film. I know I can't and I'm bloody well dying!

A year ago, I would have said I would be the last person to ask for advice on how to live your life. I put my life on the back burner for someone else for over a decade. This isn't unusual. So many of us get into relationships and lose ourselves to the other person, which is totally acceptable. It's just how much of ourselves we lose to the other person that matters. So what if you used to be a Broncos supporter and when you started dating your new boyfriend you defected to the Cowboys. This is normal and an insignificant life change. It's not like you've disowned your first-born for him. But what's not okay is when your partner starts dictating to you who you can and can't hang out with; when they start to tell you what to wear because you supposedly look like a street-walker in every second outfit you put on. So they demand that you change into an outfit of their choice. That kind of thing.

It's okay when he/she asks you to not go out with your friends tonight because they've had a shit day at work and would just love to have a night in with their partner, eating pizza and drinking a nice wine. But what's not okay is when he/she starts making excuses for you to stay home every time you are meant to be having a night out without them. You get the idea.

Yes, I'm talking about my former relationship, and a lot more happened that I'm not writing here. Of course, hindsight is 20/20, and I can now say that I would never put myself in that predicament again. I suppose that's why I am qualified to give advice about how to embrace life because for so long I didn't have one. Now that I do, even though I'm dying, I can say one thing for certain, and that's to keep those who build you up around you and get rid of those who knock you down. Why? Because at the end of the day, they are like cancers in your life unless you cut them out. Life cannot get better.

> Keep those who build you up around you and get rid of those who knock you down.

So, what is the actual advice that I give when I'm asked this question? It's pretty much what I mentioned above:

"Life is to be lived."
"Each day is a gift not an entitlement, so live it like it's your last."

"Try to laugh at least once a day."

"Hug someone every day."

"Tell someone you love them every day and tell yourself you love yourself every day."

Also, blast that idiot who repeatedly leaves the empty milk bottle in the office fridge at work. and isn't it funny that it's the same idiot who doesn't refill the paper tray in the photocopier? Make sure you publicly blast them for that one too.

Get up early one day and watch the sunrise and get home early from work one day and watch the sunset. Embrace the amazingness that is the night sky – the twinkling stars, the waning moon, the constellations and the occasional shooting star.

Don't let that person slide in front of you in the self-serve line at Woolworths. It's bad enough that you have to serve yourself, never mind letting some sneaky shithead jump the queue. Pull them up on it and make them go to the end of the queue just like the rest of us normal human beings have to.

> Embrace every day like there is no tomorrow.

Embrace every day like there is no tomorrow because that is one thing we are never promised, whether terminally ill or not, that we will wake up in the morning or make it to bed that night. We will all come to the same end at some point, so make the bits in between worth it. X

One of Lisa's biggest regrets was not making changes to her personal life long before she did. Unfortunately, it took the terminal prognosis to help her see clearly what was happening and the impact it was having on her happiness. Over the years, Lisa's self-worth had slowly dwindled until it was practically non-existent. Along with this she lost many friends, and for years the time she spent with family was limited and was always stressful as she was constantly waiting for the next problem. Unfortunately, by the time she had made major changes to her life she was either too weak or too heavily medicated to enjoy it to the full.

When Lisa first moved home, she found it extremely difficult to adapt. Peter and I couldn't understand this initially. We thought that the relief of finally being her own person and able to make her own decisions would instantly make her happy. It took us a while to understand that she had become so conditioned to living under someone else's control and having to fight for every little bit of independence. Thankfully, Lisa recognised this herself and the more time she spent at home the less we saw of her need to control. Through time life became somewhat easier for us all.

Just Because I Have Cancer Doesn't Mean...

12/07/2016

This is a sentence I use numerous times a day: "Just because I have cancer doesn't mean..."

Just because I have cancer doesn't mean I've lost my sense of humour.

Just because I have cancer doesn't mean I no longer have any interest in your life.

Just because I have cancer doesn't mean I do nothing else in my life other than cancer-related activities.

Just because I have cancer doesn't mean I don't like to look pretty and so on.

I totally get it, especially early on in the piece ... If a friend of yours has just been diagnosed with cancer, like most people, it's only natural they're going to want to talk about it. But there comes a point when we really need to start to pump the brakes on all the cancer talk. I don't mean you have to stop talking about

Just reduce the amount of C-word we use in the average conversation.

it completely. Just reduce the amount of C-word we use in the average conversation.

I love nothing more than a good old gossip, or chin wag as the more mature of us like to call it, with a girlfriend. The seedier the better. The dirtier the topic of conversation the more interested I am. Quite often, after you're diagnosed with cancer your friends can feel guilty when they talk about their seemingly minuscule problems compared to yours. No f * * * **g way. You don't get away with not telling me every last detail about the girl at work who is sleeping with your boss, even though they're both married and play poker tournaments in couples teams with each other's partners every third weekend! I live for that shit; that is the stuff that keeps me going!

I love hearing about how shitty your day at work was and then you had to go home to a sink full of dirty dishes and stinking raw chicken that's gone off because your boyfriend left it sitting in direct 35-degree sunlight all day. Now not only do you have rotten chicken smell all through your house, you also don't have dinner and it's 7.30pm. That's the stuff that distracts me from the stuff that swirls around my head 24 hours a day. Again, I live for that shit.

I HATE with every bone in my body the old 'Awww you wouldn't wanna hear about that. You've got more important things to worry about' sentence. So just a pre-warning for all of you out there: If you use the aforementioned sentence in my presence and it's directed at me, be prepared to be given the old 'Just because I have cancer doesn't make me any less of a gossip whore than I was before I had cancer' speech.

People just automatically think that as soon as pathology results come back with the word 'cancer' written on the paperwork, we become different people. It's bad enough that our own bodies are trying to kill us off, never mind our (as well-meaning, loving and adoring as they are) friends trying to kill our personalities off as well. It's like we become the boy in the bubble. We can see everything that's going on around us. We just can't quite smell it, touch it, taste it or hear it properly. We're shielded from the evils of the world, and most importantly, we're shielded from what our friends believe to be the boring bits of their lives, their boring stories, their good news bits and the list goes on. People begin to walk on eggshells around us.

"Ssssh, don't tell her that. That could be her breaking point. She has enough problems to deal with." I beg of you, give me the option as to whether your story should be told or binned. That's half the fun. I miss being able to tell you that the story you just told was shit and asking you at the end "Is that it? Sorry I thought there'd be more to it!"

Your boring, every-day, mundane stories are the bits of our lives that are so often stolen from us by cancer. That's why we need your stories. We need to live vicariously through you.

> We need to live vicariously through you.

Cancer doesn't just steal our health; it completely changes our lifestyle. If you're on active treatment such as chemo, you basically wrap yourself up in cling wrap from the beginning to the end of treatment as you have no immune system. So that little cold a little visitor caught at school can become a full-blown emergency department visit, with IVs and fevers so high you get rigors (uncontrollable shaking and feeling cold caused by a high temperature). Believe me, they're not pleasant. I've been there, got the t-shirt, twice, followed by a 7-day stay at hotel cancer ward loaded up on IV antibiotics and basically being isolated from the outside world. All because a little visitor licked the same slide the kid with the cold wiped his snotty hand on!

The trials and tribulations for those who are still curative are bad enough, such as the low immunity mentioned before. Then there's the mental side of it. They're going through the scariest scenario imaginable, so they need your mundane stories and your exciting and positive stories. They are the everyday things they are so used to having in their lives, which have been completely stripped away from them. All they're left with is a bald head and what feels like an empty soul. They're just sitting back frozen in this cancer limbo, watching the world around them whizz by functioning as normal, while they're going through their own personal hell.

Then there's me, the terminal cancer patient – the one who can't work. Let's face it, who wants an employee who could be serving a customer one minute and convulsing in pain on the shop floor the next? Many of us can't exercise, and for many people out there, exercise is their escape and therapy. Some of us can't even meditate because we can't sit in one position comfortably long enough to get into a meditative state. The drugs we're on not only drastically alter our appearance, they can also drastically alter our personalities. Personality: the one thing you think is uniquely yours and no-one but you can change. Well, you don't even have control over that. As I've mentioned before, the freedom of something as simple as driving is taken from you because of the drugs. You lose the ability to simply remain awake and concentrate during a conversation. I have micro sleeps aaaaaaaalllzzzzzzzz day long now.

I can't drink champagne like it's lemonade anymore. Subsequently, I no longer have those fun, random drunk-girl-pub-toilet conversations that I used to relish almost more than the actual night out. And then there are the big moments, the more serious ones in life ... There's a high likelihood I'm never going to get married, let alone even have another relationship. I mean someone may find an expiry date on a woman a good thing, but somehow, I don't think they're the right person for me or any self-respecting person for that matter. This means no hen's party!!!!!!!! Nope, no getting to wear the dicky bride sash and getting my own special light-up bride dick straw. No, I'm never going to own my own home. No, I'm never going to get to sail the European coast or swim in the warm waters of Bora Bora like I've always dreamt of. And probably the biggest kicker of them all (well, apart from the fact I'll probably never reach 40) ... drum roll please ... number one on the list of the things I get to miss out on because I have terminal cancer: babies of my own.

This is why it is imperative that you don't stop telling me your stories. It's so important that you keep telling me about EVERYTHING in your life, both the good and the bad! STOP censoring your life because I'm dying. You and your life may be just what's keeping me going, just like my beautiful friend who sent me a series of pictures in chronological order of her baby the other day. Such a thoughtful thing to do, especially considering the last one was of her gorgeous baby covered in her own shit. You see what type of boring life I would have if I didn't have my friends to live through vicariously. If my friend felt guilty because she could squeeze a baby out of her wing wang and I can't, I wouldn't have squirted my drink through my nose in laughter the other day when I opened that glorious picture message.

I would have continued to sit in my bubble, on the lounge, watching the rest of the world living whilst I'm slowly dying.

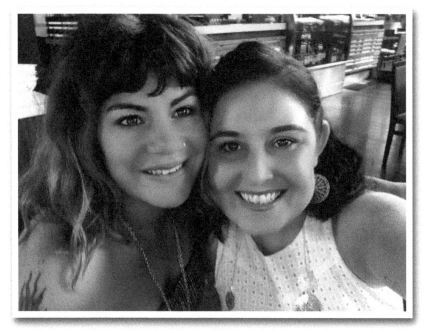

July 2016
Lisa with Constance Hall at Byron Bay for the Rafiki Mwema fundraiser.
After meeting via blogging, they remained firm friends.

How to Tell Toddlers to Teenagers You're Terminal...

19/07/2016

... and Your Time is Nearly Up

"Is your belly all better now Lisa?" This is a question I am asked daily by my two-year-old niece who's turning three in August. How do you explain to a child who is close to you, or your own children, that you have a disease that will eventually take you away from them?

Like me you may not have your own children, but that doesn't mean you aren't important to other people's children, whether they be related to you or a friend's child. If you're involved in a kid's life and you suddenly disappear, if they're old enough, they will notice your absence.

My niece Ava was born eight days before it was confirmed that my cancer had returned and that I was indeed a dead woman walking. I visited with a couple of different oncologists and the outcome of each visit, apart from one specialist, was basically the same: I would be lucky to get weeks if not months, but I certainly wouldn't be here in a year's time. I only got hope from one oncologist, and he was able to give me the confidence and the positive reinforcement that I needed so that I would persist and get as much life out of this crappy situation as possible. Months and weeks just did not sit well with me, and I have always said I just want to make it until Ava gets to big school, which would make her five. We are now nearly at three, so we are over halfway there.

For Ava's entire life I have lived with the knowledge that I am dying. I never thought I would be here a couple of months out of my niece turning three, so I didn't think I would have to consider how to broach the subjects of my illness and my imminent death with my niece. I just presumed she would be too young to understand what was going on with her aunty. Like where did all her hair go? Why is she always in the hospital and she doesn't come home with us? Why does she give herself needles? Why does Nanna give her needles in the bottom? Why does she go in the ambulance sometimes? Why is your belly so fat now, Lisa? (This is now a daily one as my belly is getting bigger by the week due to drugs.) So many questions that I never thought would be asked and need to be answered. But here we are at a point that we really need to explain to her what is going on.

Ava sees a lot of things that no adult should have to witness, never mind a toddler. A palliative care ward is scary enough for an adult to walk into, never mind a young child. A palliative ward is full of terribly sick people that are on the verge of dying. This ward is the last port of call that patients go to before saying goodbye to the world. You are surrounded by mostly elderly people who are in a terrible state. They are usually very weak, bedridden, moaning, crying, yelling out in pain, begging to die, terribly skinny ... Basically, they look like they're at death's door. This is very confronting for adults, never mind a child. But Ava takes it in her stride.

The other day my SIL (sister-in-law) Marianne was on Skype with her mum and she happened to mention that we had to wait for an ambulance, which took so long that I would've died if I was having a tumour bleed. To this Ava piped up in the background and asked, "Is Lisa dying?" Marianne was taken aback because she didn't think firstly that Ava would be listening because she was happily playing in the background. And secondly, she didn't expect her two-year-old child to be asking about her aunty dying. Marianne responded "Of course not. The doctors fixed her." But Marianne realised that we really do need to explain to Ava what is actually going on. We can't just keep saying Lisa has a sore belly.

Children are not stupid or oblivious to what is going on around them. They sense distress, and when they get to a certain age like Ava is now, they become inquisitive. They may not always understand the answer, but they certainly know how to ask the questions.

> Children are not stupid or oblivious to what is going on around them.

Another thing I have realised is that many of the cartoons and movies that children are watching feature death. Look at *Bambi*, *Babe*, *The Lion King* and even *Toy Story 3*, when they're all in the incinerator facing death and basically just sit back, waiting to die. Luckily, they're saved, but once again kids are faced with the reality that death is a part of life. Books that kids read expose them to death from an early age, like Harry Potter. He loses his parents and many other pivotal people in his life. What I think is that kids just don't understand the reality of it.

Ava has found me writhing in pain on the toilet floor and had to alert my dad. This is no sight any child should have to see, but this is Ava's reality, like it is for so many other children out there. Ava has spent more time in hospital rooms and wards than she has had hot dinners. Ava likes to alcohol-wipe my injection site before injections, and if I'm not at home she presumes I'm at the doctor's or hospital. She asks if my belly is better every day, and she dresses up in her Doc McStuffins doctor's coat and knows exactly how to listen to my chest and tells me to cough.

So what would my advice be to those out there who must inform their own child/children, or a child in their life, that an important person in their life is dying? It all depends on their age. Although Ava is very perceptive and absorbs information like a sponge (Seriously, you drop the s-word in front of her and she'll dob on you quicker than a Real Housewife of New Jersey will flip a table. She certainly likes to tell on you; Aunty Lisa gets in trouble a lot!), we have to remember that she is still only a two-year-old little girl. Although she behaves and acts like an eight-year-old, we sometimes forget she is still only a toddler.

Ava and I have gone out at dusk and watched beautiful sunsets. I've pointed out the moon and the stars to her when it gets dark, so she has developed an affection for and interest in the night sky. At some point, Ava's mum and dad will start to discuss the fact that all the stars in the sky are loved ones that have passed away and their job is to look after their families at night. So when I finally pass, a star will be appointed 'Aunty Lisa' and it will be explained that I am no longer here on earth, but I am up in the sky looking down every night over Ava and our family. I will keep everyone safe at night time when she is in bed. (I love this idea because so many kids get nightmares and are scared of the dark and knowing someone in the sky is protecting them throughout the night will help them sleep. Well, this is what I'm hoping for anyway, and I'm sure Ava's parents are hoping for the same result.) The next step will be that Ava can go out and speak to Aunty Lisa (the star in the sky) and tell her any secrets, stories or how school was – anything she wants to talk about. She can talk to me in the sky. This gives me comfort, knowing that my memory will be kept alive.

When it comes to older children, I believe honesty is your best policy. I have witnessed a young family, the mum would have been in her mid-30s, and they spoke openly in front of the kids (probably 8 and 13) about her terminal bowel cancer and her terminal prognosis. Don't treat kids with kid gloves. Treat them as they deserve to be treated, as young adults that are entitled to know that their mother or father is not going to be around forever and, unfortunately, their ending will be sooner than most. You have to allow children the chance to come to terms with the fact that they are going to lose a parent, and you need to give them the chance to show that parent how much they truly love them and how much they mean to them. Let's face it, kids have a habit of fighting with their parents. How many times do you hear a kid yelling out that they hate their parent?

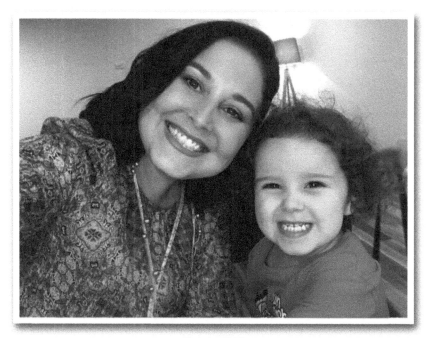

18 July 2016
Lisa and Ava at Ava's home. Say 'Cheese'!

So you need to let them know that you have limited time, so they can enjoy whatever time they have with you. Imagine them going to bed yelling at you because they were in a pivotal moment playing *World of Warcraft* and you're making them go to bed, and they hate you and wish Taylor's parents were their parents. And they hope you disappear in the middle of the night because you're simply the worst parents EVER!!!! Then you go to bed and don't wake up. Is that fair to your child?

I get it. I'm not a parent, so where do I get off giving advice about something I have absolutely no knowledge of? You're right, I don't have the right. But I do have the right to an opinion and this is mine You don't have to listen to it. You don't have to use it. I'm just putting it out there into the universe because that's what I do. All I want for those poor kids who are going to lose a parent or person close to them, no matter how old they are, is to have some closure and some level of understanding and acceptance before they go through probably the most horrendous thing a child could ever go through.

Here are just a few websites and links that can help children and adults who are dealing with cancer and bereavement in their lives. I have supplied some web addresses for Australia, the US and United Kingdom. But if you google you can find many different agencies that can help.

Australia

www.cancer.org.au

www.cancercouncil.com.au/1374/uncategorized/when-a-parent-has-cancer-4

www.bereavementcare.com.au

www.feelthemagic.org.au

www.grief.org.au

www.kidshelp.com.au

USA

www.kidskonnected.org

www.cancer.net/coping-with-cancer/managing-emotions/grief-and-loss/helping-grieving-children-and-teenagers

UK

www.riprap.org.uk

www.winstonswish.org.uk

www.childbereavementuk.org/support/families

Throughout the cancer journey people will make mistakes; I know I did. How can you not? All you can do is your best. However, where Ava is concerned, I think we somehow did well as a family preparing her for what lay ahead. I'm not sure if that was because Ava was who she was, or if we actually did make the best decisions through pure good luck.

One thing we did not want was for Ava to wake one morning to be told Lisa had gone to heaven and for her to have no understanding at all of what we were on about. During the last few months of Lisa's life, it was evident that her body could not take much more pain and suffering. Although her heart was strong and her determination unbreakable, her body was weakening fast. We began discussing Lisa becoming an angel with Ava, and how eventually at night she would be the brightest star in the sky watching over us all to keep us safe.

At first, Ava was adamant she did not want Lisa to go to heaven. She wanted to be able to kiss and hug her at night. It was heart-breaking to hear, but we continued with these discussions by explaining that Lisa would no longer be in pain and would not have to have painful injections and lots of medicine. As much as she never fully accepted the idea of Lisa leaving, she knew it was going to happen. She would ask questions. Some we didn't know how to answer, but we somehow got through them. One thing we learnt quite early in the piece was to be consistent with what we were telling her, otherwise it would cause confusion and could lead to her disbelieving what she was being told.

Looking back, Ava's reaction was no different to any of ours. We knew what lay ahead and we didn't want to believe it. Even after Ava was told what she needed to know, she spoke of it rarely. Like us all she could pretend it wasn't happening until it happened. When push comes to shove that's how we all got by, not thinking past today.

I think it is important to mention that this never impacted on Lisa and Ava's close relationship. Ava had no fear on the days Lisa's pain levels were high. She seemed to know that the medication given would take a while to kick in, and once it did it was back to play time again. Just because there was no rough-and-tumble play didn't mean there was no fun. There was lots of singing, dancing, make-up sessions (more like clown sessions) and make-believe storytelling and acting it out. They both got so much out of it. On the days when Lisa was feeling up to it, she would do crafts with Ava. She wanted to make the most of their time together. Obviously, near the end this was impossible. But when up to it Lisa would call Ava up to her room and they'd watch a movie.

As strange as it may seem, it was easier for Ava to cope with Lisa's condition as she was practically born into it. Medication, syringes, blood, pain drivers, wheelchairs and even visits to palliative care were all normal to Ava. I believe our greatest challenges will come now in getting Ava to understand that a hospital visit to someone she knows doesn't mean a hospital stay or a long-term terminal illness. But we have no regrets in how we have handled this situation. In fact, I feel immense pride when I think of it.

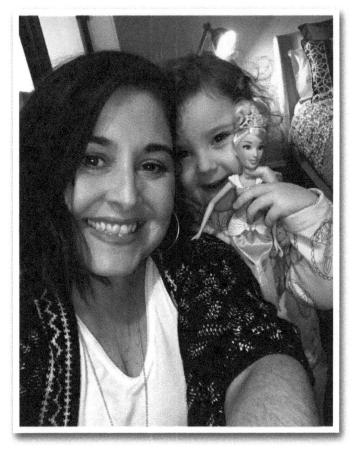

June 2016
Lisa and Ava at home taking playtime selfies!

Doctor/Patient Relationships and Blurred Lines

23/07/2016

So, this week I was totally blindsided. I was dumped by my doctor. I know, right. Who gets dumped by their doctor?

I totally get it if they move practices or quit or retire. But if you move around the corner from your old house and your doctor tells you they can no longer do house visits and give you the care you need or deserve, all because you've moved four streets away from your old house, well, no I don't get it.

What I do get, though, is that you have a gorgeous family you have to get home to in the evenings, and you don't need to be stopping in to visit me to take my blood pressure. That's eating into your precious time with your kids and family; I totally get it. But you gave me your mobile number; you were always contactable. You were so caring, and your service was above reproach. I truly believed we were more than the doctor/patient relationship; I thought we were more like friends.

I feel like I'm going through a divorce. My current doctor has already recommended a new, more local doctor and referred me onto them, like I've signed up to a doctor/patient matching website. 'Have you recently been dumped by your doctor? Do you feel like your old doctor didn't understand you? Never fear, we here at eHarmony Doctors will find you the perfect match.' This is probably sounding ludicrous to you as you read it, but for those of you who have a chronic illness or health issues that require regular visits to doctors or specialists, you'll get it.

This is not the first time I've confused my doctor/patient relationship for more than that. You see, you spend so much time with these people that sometimes the lines can become a bit blurred. Just because your specialist calls you at 10pm with results, ends their text messages with emojis and hugs you at the end of appointments does not mean they think you are or ever will be friends. (Okay, maybe the hug's more me than them, but they don't have to hug back!)

I've had a specialist actually say to me once – when my cancer had returned and it was terminal and we knew I'd be lucky to have weeks – that this is why he doesn't become close to patients. It's too difficult when things like this happen and he can't handle it.

I think I've probably secretly fallen in love with most of my medical team at some point in my treatment. When you're in hospital for a month at a time and you wake up every morning to your specialist or registrar, who is really lovely, caring, attentive, funny and you know that if you went into cardiac arrest at any moment, they could sort that shit out pronto, it's attractive. You can become attracted. I've had more than one or two dreams of one or more of my specialists, registrars and ED doctors over the years. In fact, I still believe if I was single, one particular one would have asked me to marry him years ago.

What is it about doctors? Is it because we tend to have this God-complex-thing going on about them, you know like we have about firemen, soldiers, policemen, men in uniforms or positions of power? As soon as we see a man with a helmet, our loins start to ache! Imagine if you were seeing this person day in day out, it's no wonder patients fall in love or get confused and think their professional relationship is a friendship.

Well, I'm here to tell you, it's not. And if it is, it's probably committing some sort of illegal act. I have no idea what the rules/laws are when it comes to doctor/patient relationships, but I imagine they are not looked upon favourably.

> They are your doctor, not your partner and not your best friend.

So my Fabulous Rockstars, if you're starting to go all gooey-eyed at the thought of seeing your specialist at your next appointment, or you're paying more attention to what you're wearing and your make-up before your next appointment, just remember they are your doctor, not your partner and not your best friend. They are there to heal you not hug you, and at the end of the day if you take your rose-coloured glasses off and take a real good look at them, there's a very high chance that they look more like *ER's* Dr Mark Greene (Anthony Edwards) than Dr Doug Ross (George Clooney).

Take it from a patient scorned, keep your patient/doctor relationship professional. I promise, you'll thank me in the long run. And please remember to take this blog in the way it was intended – tongue in cheek.

Stay Fabulous, Rockstars.

And remember, keep your hands off your doctor's stethoscopes.

As much as Lisa jokes about losing her GP, it really did knock her about for a while. She had built a strong relationship with her doctor, who was really amazing. She went out of her way to ensure both Lisa and I were supported at the most difficult of times. I do think there was a bit of blurred lines for Lisa regarding her relationship with her GP. The GP was quite young and was able to connect with Lisa because of this. Because she was terminal at 34, Lisa did get special treatment not always available to everyone, more home visits and so on. I think that because of this, Lisa interpreted it as friendship. In fact, she made mention of this during her palliative care visits, and I think it was recognised that Lisa was maybe misinterpreting the purpose of their relationship.

As Lisa said herself, it is easily done. There were times when Lisa would only see family and her doctor as she wasn't fit to leave the house. Thankfully, the GP that her doctor recommended was just as lovely, who once again was absolutely amazing with Lisa and all of us. We all became extremely fond of her, and she has remained our family GP.

Does it Matter if You're Scarred for Life if You're Dying?

28/07/2016

Does it matter if you're scarred for life if you're dying? My answer is a resounding yes. Initially when I was operated on, I wasn't fazed by my abdominal scarring. It was only one neat straight line from my belly button to the side and four small keyhole scars. They were my battle wounds – proof I'd fought and survived. But with each surgery that followed, the more complex the scarring became. When I say complex, I do mean uglier, more obvious – less Joaquin Phoenix obvious scarring and more Seal, the Kiss from a Rose singer, scarring. Yes, I know he is a fabulous singer with a voice as smooth as silk, and he scored a supermodel for a wife, but the poor guy has got obvious facial scarring. At the end of the day, like with me, the scarring was completely out of his control.

Life is so fragile, but some people have the ability to keep treating their bodies like a garbage bin with no consequences. They continually put pretend food like McDonalds in their body and have perfect cholesterol. They smoke a pack a day and have lungs like a cheetah (they have a really high lung capacity because of the speed they run), and they're the ones who still have a sunbed in their attic and have never had a questionable mole, the ones who base jump, parkour, bull ride, bull run and volcano board (yes, this is a real thing). The list of idiotic, life-threatening activities that one can risk their lives doing is endless. Meanwhile, there is a sterile room full of people somewhere, sitting in recliners and hooked up to IVs having poisonous chemicals pumped into their veins to give themselves an extra chance at survival.

My scarring used to be something I would show off proudly when I thought I was cured. Then I had three more surgeries, and the fact that I'm no longer curable, the scars have become more of a constant reminder that I am dying rather than a sign of strength. Every time I take my clothes off in the bathroom, there they are in the mirror. When I lift up my top to let the nurse access my pain med access point, there it is. When I go for a swim, there it is. I see it every day, and every day it whispers loudly in my head, "Oh yeah, don't forget you're dying."

> Tomorrow I will embrace my scarring again.

Scars are not something to be ashamed of. You might think from what I have said above that they are something to be hidden and not embraced. But that couldn't be further from my opinion. It's simply that I am having one of those days that I hate everything about my body, and because I have a blog, I blog about it. So please don't take this

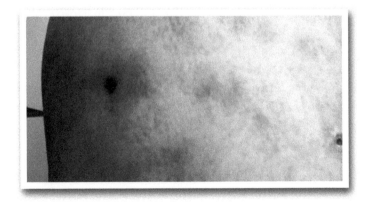

as a 'hide your scars' blog. I say be proud of your scars. It's just that today I am bloated and sore, and the more bloated I am the more prominent my scarring. Tomorrow I will embrace my scarring again, but the one thing that will never change is the fact that they are unfortunately the daily reminder that I'm dying. I could choose to look at them as my daily reminder that I am fighting. Maybe that's how I should start to look at them: fighting scars.

As the person that spent most time with Lisa, I know that the scars were not a major issue for her. However, I do believe that the bloating and inability to fit into her clothes had a big impact on her and how she felt about her body. Hence, why the scarring was being mentioned. Throughout Lisa's late teens and her twenties, Lisa was extremely self-critical of her hair, her face, her thighs and the list goes on. We could never understand it. All we could see was a beautiful, young woman who was always immaculate and always took pride in her appearance. As the cancer and treatments progressed, Lisa yearned for the face and body of that woman in her twenties. At times it felt like she was grieving for her old self. It was heart-breaking to watch her feel such despair. As far as Lisa was concerned cancer was going to take her life, but why did it have to take everything else in the process?

These are the physical and mental changes that not a lot of people talk about openly during the cancer journey. Yes, saving the person's life is the first priority, and Lisa understood that. But it doesn't stop anyone from struggling mentally to accept how they have changed. Although Lisa resisted counselling, I often tried to encourage her to have it because I think it may have helped her prepare for these changes better.

Chemo Refresher

10/08/2016

So I met this lovely woman just over a month ago called Hayley, and she asked to interview me for a local magazine. Of course, I was all excited and felt all special that I was doing my first legitimate meet-in-a-coffee-shop-be-asked-questions-maybe-get-a-photo proper interview.

Hayley arrived, and we began to chat back and forth. All the while I was thinking *Is she ever going to ask me a question? This isn't going how I pictured it. It's more like a chat than an interview.* As we exchanged stories and I talked all things terminal cancer, Hayley dropped a bomb. She too may have cancer and would be finding out, after a biopsy in the following days, exactly what she was dealing with.

Excuse me while I choke on my English Breakfast tea, black with two raw sugars. What the actual fuck? You reach out to me to do an interview on cancer and then find out you have some sort of breast cancer. Cue my anthem Alanis Morrissette's *Ironic* because this shit doesn't happen in real life, except that it did.

Hayley went in for a biopsy a few days later. Fast forward to today and she is one boob short and bald. I've just returned home from visiting her whilst she was getting her second cycle of chemo, celebrating her 29th birthday with a homemade cake that her mum lovingly made for her, her chemo nurses and her chemo buddy for the day, her sister Lauren.

For any of you out there that have had chemo before, you'll understand exactly what I am about to say. On the car trip into the hospital to visit her, I started to feel nauseated at the thought of going into that room again with pale, bald, sickly looking people and the stench of chemo floating through the air. You're probably thinking this sounds terribly selfish of me thinking of myself while she's going through this horrible ordeal. But people who have had chemo often get 'chemo anxiety'. They get it when they see needles and have to be cannulated or give blood. I've even been told of a woman projectile vomiting in the street when she came face to face with her oncologist from 20 years prior. I used to get it every time I had to return to my oncology ward to be scanned every three months. I haven't had it since, so I was surprised when I started to get those horrible chemo nausea-like symptoms in the car.

As I sat next to Hayley and Lauren as Hayley was being cannulated and that vile poison started to pulse through her veins, I had to push down the vomit in my throat. I was back in the chair on my first day of chemo, when I had no idea what lay ahead of me and thought in the first few hours, *This shit's easy. What does everyone complain about? I got this. Chemo's my bitch!* Six hours later, with my head in a sick bag, feeling like I'd just been hit by a bus, I realised I was chemo's bitch.

I left Hayley this afternoon, and all that's been going through my head since are thoughts like the horrible pain and headaches I got when I started to lose my hair. YES, IT HURTS!!!!! I shaved it within days of feeling the pain of it dragging on my scalp, as though I had weights tied into it. I couldn't deal with it on top of the horrendous sickness, tiredness and feeling of death that hung over me.

As soon as I got home, I had to get Mum to inject me with a sickness med. As I sit here and type, I am feeling as sick as a dog again. So whilst I bitch and moan about the way I feel at the thought of chemo, let's spare a thought for Hayley and the thousands of other men and women who at this exact moment have their heads in the toilet and know that in a couple of weeks they have to face up to it again. I salute you!

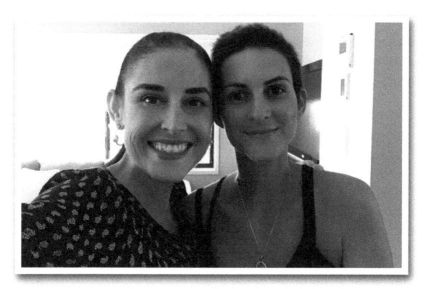

17 February 2017
Lisa and Hayley Walker – a good friend and journalist who was on her own cancer journey – at home in Springfield Lakes, QLD.

Once she had committed to helping someone else through their journey, there was no going back.

I used to wonder what people meant when they said the treatment is worse than the illness. I'd think that's impossible. But when it comes to chemo it's so true, some chemos more than others. I remember that day well. The drive in was more nerve-wracking than usual. Because of Lisa's tumour pain driving was never enjoyable. She would feel every lump and bump in the road. I half-expected Lisa to tell me to turn around, she was that anxious. But that was Lisa. Once she had committed to helping someone else through their journey, there was no going back.

I was so worried about what impact this would have on Lisa's already fragile state of mind, and I could fully understand where she was coming from. I still get butterflies in the tummy when I have to go near the hospital. The memories come flashing back one after the other. If I'm in the shopping centre and someone passes me with no hair or eyebrows, my mind automatically goes into overdrive, and it takes me a while to compose myself. So this day was never going to be easy for Lisa.

Lisa was extremely pale when leaving the hospital, and it was a very quiet journey home, which was highly unusual. I knew that Lisa was shaken, and once I gave her a sickness injection, she went to her room to hide out until she felt up to talking. I think, along with chemo anxiety, there was also a feeling of hurt and disappointment. Lisa had endured so many treatments, each with their own cruel after-effects, and all in vain. I know she wanted the best for Hayley, but it didn't stop her hurting and wishing.

Hayley and I have remained close since Lisa's passing. I'm so pleased to say she is now in remission and has really changed her focus in life. Art has always been her passion, and she has left work to pursue this passion. She's doing extremely well. I know Lisa will be looking down on her with pride.

Do I envy the fact that Hayley is doing so well yet Lisa is no longer with us? Not at all. Cancer not only changed Lisa, it changed us all in some ways. Prior to Lisa's illness I was like any other mother. I noticed every single thing that was going on in my own family circle, but I'd hardly notice anything outside that circle. Now I seem to notice so much more of what's going on around me. I see someone in a wheelchair looking ill and my heart hurts for them. I instantly wonder if I should go over and offer help. I see someone with a port protruding from their chest and I contemplate asking them how their treatment is going. I want to know all about their cancer journey, and I want to offer them help.

But the reality is I don't speak to them. I don't offer them help because I just can't, yet. The best I can do for those I see is to hope and pray to God that their journey has a far happier ending than ours.

> "I opened two gifts this
> morning – my eyes."
>
> –Author unknown

Family Getaway

13/08/2016

We just had our two-year anniversary family weekend. This was our third mini break on the coast since being told in 2014 that I would be lucky to make it to Christmas. And here we are, a couple of weeks off celebrating my third bonus Christmas.

I was really looking forward to our little family mini break. I was especially excited to see my brother's reaction to the hotel we were staying at. I bought six bottles of champagne that were on sale, and I thought I was going to have the hangover of all hangovers. But what I had imagined and what was the reality of the weekend were two completely different things.

From Ava being obsessed with the bidet in the master bathroom and me catching her sneaking a sip of water directly from it and washing her hands in it, to the air conditioning not working all weekend and all of us sweating like a whore in church, it was a very different weekend to what it would have been BC (Before Cancer). BC I would have been singing and dancing on a table before Beyoncé even got to the second verse of *Single Ladies*, and three bottles of champagne would be down before she got to the third verse. But things are different now.

Sometimes I wonder if it actually is a cancer thing that has caused this rapid decline in party animal, or if it is an age thing. It's a confusing age, 34. Ten years ago at 34 you were more likely to be married, popping your third kid out and mortgaged to the hilt. But now I see so many of my female friends on Facebook being single and partying it up. Are they actually enjoying themselves or is it just a facade they put on for Facebook? God, I could think of nothing worse than dancing at some nightclub until the ugly lights come on and then moving onto the Sunday sessions after a few hours' sleep. Give me a Christmas movie and a take-away any day.

I still wouldn't change our low-key weekend for the world. Alcohol does not make the weekend; it's the people who do. We made memories, and that's what matters. The love and the laughter we shared this weekend will remain in the corners of our hearts and minds forever. You don't have to go to some fancy hotel to make lasting memories either. The hotel is just a little bonus.

I was in bed by 9.30pm every night and didn't open one bottle of the six champagnes I bought. I probably only drank five glasses of champagne over the four days, and my pain and tiredness were overwhelming. But just knowing that all your family are in the same place is a really comforting thought.

Ava loved the whole three days. I thought she'd get there, run around excited for a minute and then start to complain about being bored. But she LOVED her 'holiday house'. She eagerly ran around the hotel room showing Grando and Nanna the pool, the big bath and the TV that was hidden in the wooden cabinet. It was like Christmas for her, and anytime we left the room, she'd ask to go back to our holiday house. I thought we'd have the hardest time getting her to go home, but she said good-bye to the pool, literally, and asked, "Can we come back to our holiday house again?"

"Of course we can sweetie ... of course we can..." Another one of those promises I've made to her that I really can't promise to keep.

Anyone out there who has, like myself, been gifted the worst Christmas present ever — I'm talking worse than the ugliest Christmas sweater ever made ... the gift of terminal cancer — I highly recommend making the effort and spending some special time with your immediate family. They will appreciate those memories more than any other gift you could possibly give.

So here we are back home, back to reality. I was hoping I accidentally had left my lethargy and nausea in the hotel room along with my phone charger. But it unfortunately seems to have followed me home. The sneaky little bastard is as hard to shake as a black van full of martial arts experts following you in a Jacki Chan movie.

It's so cliché, but life is exactly what you make of it. I could have easily cancelled our weekend away; believe me the thought crossed my mind more than once. But I figured a bed is a bed, and if I have to spend the weekend in one, it may as well be in the hotel. That way I was not letting my family down by cancelling. Ava would have been heartbroken, and I couldn't be the cause of that. The sadness on that little girl's face would have killed me.

So I put my big girl pants on and made myself go. Although I'm as tired as Geordie Shore's fake tan application assistant, I would do it all again tomorrow just to see my niece's face at the sight of the pool, my brother's and dad's excitement at the free sparkling wine in the foyer — they don't even drink the stuff, but free alcohol is free alcohol and they certainly made the most of it — my mum actually taking a minute to herself relaxing by the pool and my sister-in-law not answering phone calls from work every hour. It's amazing that a hotel an hour's drive away can feel like a whole other world. It gave us all a break from cancer for a few days. It's as if it didn't exist, and that's a wonderful gift you can give a family that faces the thought of death every day — a break from reality.

With every Christmas that goes by, I wonder how and when I will die.

This year has been full of ups and downs, Emergency Department visits, ICU admissions, palliative ward admissions, lots of pain and extreme tiredness, pain relief, radiation, immunotherapy trials, nausea and regurgitation. I've spent lots of time with those I love, friends and family from near and far. Although the year has been harder than easier, I go to bed every night

> I honestly
> feel so
> lucky when
> I open my
> eyes.

thanking God that I'm still alive, and when I wake in the morning, I thank him again for keeping me going through the night. I honestly feel so lucky when I open my eyes that I get this feeling of excitement akin to a kid on Christmas morning. My heart literally skips a beat.

Another family trip notch on our belt, and here's to us celebrating the same anniversary next year.

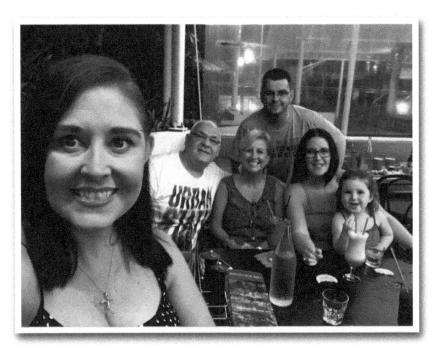

4 December 2016
Lisa, Peter, Geraldine, Steven, Marianne and Ava having a
family dinner at Palazzo Versace Hotel, Gold Coast.

We had an aunt come to visit us with my mum back in 2015. My Aunt Vera had never been to Australia nor had she seen our family for quite a while.

So as you can imagine, she was so excited and really enjoyed her time in Oz. Reading this blog always makes me think of Vera. She left Australia in September, and in January she was diagnosed with a brain tumour. By June we lost her to the disease.

During her time with us, she was in awe of Lisa and the courage she demonstrated. She couldn't understand how Lisa could get back up after so many knock downs even though her pain was merciless. Since my aunt's passing, I often thought of the two different cancer journeys. My aunt's was fast and cruel, and Lisa's was long, painful and relentless. I have asked myself many times which of the two cancer journeys were worse, and I've never come up with the answer as one was as cruel as the other.

Although our family break was not perfect, we considered it a good thing. It was a different environment, there was no need to cook and the cleaning was taken care of. To us (well, to me) that was luxury at that specific time. But more than that it was time spent together as a family. Somehow everyday frustrations were left at home. We were so grateful just to be able to get away, the rest was inconsequential.

This is probably the difference between a long and short terminal diagnosis. It's not the level of pain nor the amount of trauma it causes but the ability to make the most of every opportunity possible to spend time with loved ones. As Lisa would say, "Make hay when the sun shines". If Lisa could get out of bed and make it to the beach, she did. And if she couldn't, she would sit up in bed with the curtains pushed back and enjoy watching the ocean whilst listening to the waves crashing down.

> Make hay when the sun shines.

I was really concerned about this trip as Lisa was struggling before we left, but there was no way she would cancel. As much as Ava's heart was set on it, so was Lisa's. We will always treasure these ad hoc breaks away; the memories we made were priceless.

I often say to my friends, "Don't wait for a reason to get together as a family; just do it". The reality is we all get side-tracked by life. We get busy, but we

185

also get complacent, thinking *There is always going to be tomorrow*. As much as I promised myself that I would never again take anything for granted, and that I'd make the most of every moment, we have slowly slipped into our old ways. Every now and again, however, I stop and smell the roses. I try to remind myself of what we still have, and I try not to dwell on what we have lost.

Dear Life

16/08/2016

You gave me moments in time that I shall not forget — memories that are engraved in my mind and the minds of my family and friends for eternity. The gifts of joy and love that you have given are plentiful and infinite, and for that reason I am grateful for the life I have had. Sure, it might not be the easiest of lives ever lived. We've certainly had our ups and downs. But I hope that when my time comes, my loved ones will remember the good times you gave us rather than the bad times.

Life, you are a fickle friend. One day we are besties and the next we are mortal enemies. I never know what to expect from you. Will today be a pain-free, fight-free, fun-filled day or will it be a pain-filled, bedridden, emotional roller coaster of a day? Life, why can't you just be predictable? I know there are people out there who would say a predictable life is a boring life, a life unfulfilled. But for me, and for many others out there suffering like myself, one thing we would love in life would be predictability.

Just imagine going to bed and setting an alarm Monday to Friday for the same time, and then getting up in the morning, getting ready, eating breaky, hopping in the car, sitting in horrendous traffic whilst listening to your favourite music, bitching and moaning about traffic in between singing the chorus like you're a real fucking rockstar and not giving a shit that the person in the car next to you is looking at you as if you're Bert Newton without his wig on (Aussies know that look) and getting to work ten minutes late. You're sitting at your desk typing monotonously and constantly glancing at your phone, counting down the hours until home time when you get back in your car, sit in the same traffic in the opposite direction, get home, make dinner, watch the news and have a glass of wine. You go to bed and do it all again. Oh how sweet predictability would taste.

For those of you who hate predictability, I totally get it. There's even a saying dedicated to it: Familiarity breeds contempt. But if you lived our life of unpredictability, you'd probably beg for your predictable life back.

Life, the days you give me extreme pain, the days when my body becomes so contorted and cramped that my carer has to massage my limbs back into normality ... Why do you like to gift me these days on days that I'm meant to be going out with a friend? Or when I'm on holiday and you think it's fun to give me a tumour bleed, so I spend more time in the hospital than I do in the hotel? Oh you are a fickle friend.

Life, how do you choose who is to live and who is to die? What prerequisites must one have to escape the prematurely dying group? Why do some live to 90 whilst others live to nine? Where is the fairness in that? Do you do these things so that we 'learn' from them? Are these things meant to make us better, stronger people? Quite frankly, I'd rather be a weaker person and not experience these things in life that are meant to make us stronger.

Life, are you and God friends? Is there a connection between what happens to us in life and what God wants to happen in life? Who's the boss: God or you, Life?

> Who's the boss: God or you, Life?

Like good old Forrest Gump said, "Life is like a box of chocolates. You never know what you're gonna get". Well, sorry Forrest, any box of chocolates you buy has a fucking list of exactly what each chocolate contains. Why can't Life have a list of exactly what it's going to contain, so we know what to expect?

Life, you've had me dying for years. Why couldn't you just tell me an exact date, so I can stop living you in limbo, not knowing day from day if it will be my last?

Life, you are the greatest gift of all, but Jesus Christ, there are some days you feel more like a pair of socks at Christmas rather than a piece of jewellery.

Fabulous Rockstars, I hope that your Life is the gift you asked Santa for and not a pair of socks.

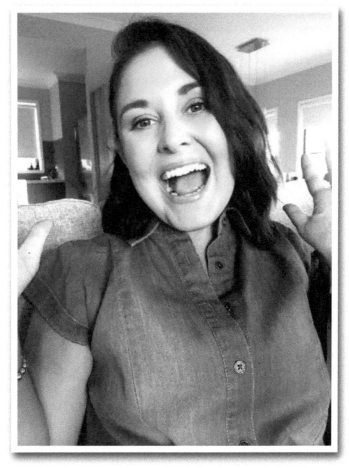

16 August 2016
Lisa

I remember many times wishing life could just be normal, even for a day. If I could only go shopping without worrying that my phone would ring with another emergency ... If I could just arrange to go to lunch with a friend without having to think twice about anything or anyone else ...

That would be the perfect day. Looking back now, all these things are so inconsequential, so unimportant. Why was it such a big deal at the time? Now that I have all the time in the world to do these things, they do not hold the same level of enjoyment I imagined they would.

Unlike Lisa, I thank God that we do not know what lies ahead. If someone had told me back in January 2012 what lay ahead of us, and how difficult it would be, I am confident I would have suffered a breakdown at the very thought of it. I firmly believe that innocence is bliss. There is time enough to worry about things as and when they happen, never mind knowing and dreading what lay ahead. I remember the frustration we would feel at not knowing what to expect, and when people would ask us the dreaded "How long have they given Lisa?" truth be told, no-one knew.

The cancer was rare, although we knew it was sarcoma. This type of sarcoma had never been seen before, so everything was trial and error. There were many times we were told that Lisa would be gone within the next month or two. But not only were they dealing with this type of cancer for the first time, they were also dealing with Lisa for the first time. Her strength and determination to live as long as humanly possible was unbelievable and heart-breaking. Lisa was a shell of her former self.

I am unsure if it was Lisa's will to live that kept her going or her fear of death.

To this day I am unsure if it was Lisa's will to live that kept her going or her fear of death.

The Second Most Important Man in My Life

23/08/2016

Tonight, I asked my brother if he would do my eulogy at my funeral, not if he would do a speech at my wedding, not if he'd be godfather to my child. No, my eulogy. He was somewhat taken aback by this request. You see, I forgot that I had already thought about this and let it marinate for a few days, but this was the first he was hearing of it.

189

I mentioned to him that neither Mum or Dad particularly wanted to do it, because they didn't know how they would feel on the day and whether emotionally they would be up to it. My brother responded, "Well, I don't know how I'll be on the day." To be honest that took me aback a bit. You see, I just figured Steven being Steven will front up on the day, chat to a few people, introduce himself to a few randoms, tell them a few awkward or inappropriate funeral jokes, and then take his seat at the front of the chapel and be his normal stoic, unemotional self. Then when he has a minute at home by himself, he might have a bit of a cry, pull himself together and then be what he thinks he is: the rock of the family. The one who has the answers to all the hard questions. The one who has the shoulder for everyone else to cry on.

I love my brother more than life itself, and I would honestly throw myself in front of a car to save his life. Yes, even before I was dying I would have done this. I always wanted to be besties with my bro. We moved to Australia at the ages of eight and five, Steven being the youngest. I loved holding Steven's hand; he hated it, especially in public. You see I was never an outgoing kid. I didn't make friends easily, so for me Steven was like a built-in friend. He couldn't reject me because he was family. But no, that didn't stop him.

I was always in awe of Steven's ability to make friends when he was a kid. It didn't matter where we would go, whether it be the McDonald's playground or in the dentist's waiting room, Steven always managed to make a friend. I just didn't have that skill.

We fought and fought our way through our teenage years. We must have driven Mum and Dad nuts. So when my brother went back to Ireland with the parentals, we grew apart. By the time they moved back, he had his long-term girlfriend and he was a man. So we had grown even further apart. We still lived in different states and would see each other a couple of times a year.

Then the Big C came and Steven being Steven put his Mr Fix-it hat on and googled every treatment, every surgeon, every hospital and every statistic. It made him feel like he had some control over something that in fact was out of all our control. His mantra became 'Plan for the worst, hope for the best'. I heard that saying more times than I've had enemas, and as we all know, many an enema I have had. I think it was as much of a wake-up call for him as it was for everyone else.

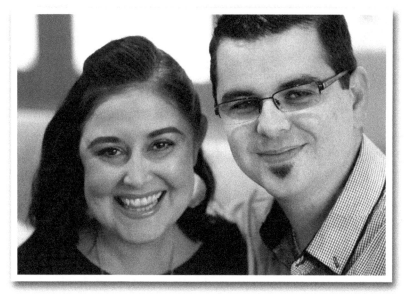

23 June 2016
Lisa and Steven at home. "I love my brother more than life itself." – Lisa

Steven and I know we both love each other. I want him to realise that I think he is one of the smartest people I know. I want him to know that we don't need to compete for our parents like we did when we were kids. Most of all I wish that he knew that my love for him, although it seems conditional, is in actual fact unconditional.

And remember, Steven, if I do come back as a ghost, your house will be my first visit. And Marianne? I promise to call ahead.

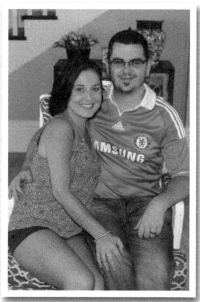

16 February 2016
Lisa and Steven at Broadbeach, Gold Coast, at the end of a girls' weekend away. Steven had arrived to pick up Marianne and Ava.

Lisa and Steven were quite different, even as children. Lisa was strong-willed and in control. Steven on the other hand was softer as a child. He needed a lot more mothering and nurturing. As time went by and Steven became a little more independent, Lisa wanted to continue to mother him, and he was having none of it. This led to many screaming matches and fights. They were constantly at each other's throats. But no matter how much they'd fight throughout the day, I'd creep into their rooms at night to check on them and Lisa was always in Steven's bed with her arm around him. It was hard to believe it was the same two children.

The fighting and arguing continued into their teens. Lisa wanted to smother Steven in hugs and kisses, but Steven didn't want a bar of it. Inevitably this would result in another argument. Even as young adults Lisa always wanted that closeness. Personal space would mean nothing to her and Steven was the exact opposite. Lisa just couldn't get her head around this and misinterpreted it as Steven not caring. However, this couldn't have been further from the truth. When Lisa was diagnosed with cancer, Steven took it as hard as the rest of us, For the first time in a long time, we could see him wearing his heart on his sleeve. He had to believe she would beat this. It was the only way he could function. Unfortunately, when the cancer metastasised, he continued to believe Lisa would be cured, and this brought further frustration to their relationship.

Lisa wanted Steven to understand that she was dying, and Steven wanted Lisa to stay strong and have faith that a cure would be found. This created a distance between them. As much as they remained as close as possible during the cancer journey, there was always that differing opinion lurking between them. For all the fighting and arguing that had taken place when they were growing up, Steven was the same as the rest of us though. Each time there was an emergency or a negative test result, he was devastated.

I will never forget the week of Lisa's passing. She had finally accepted the fact that she had nothing left to fight with and would never leave palliative care again. Although completely drugged and at times incoherent, she wanted to say some lasting words to each of us. At this point it became clear how much she had always loved Steven and how much faith she had in him to take care of her Dad and I in years to come whilst also being the best husband and dad he could be. This was a massive thing for Steven as Lisa had previously aired her concerns regarding her Dad and I during retirement. He now felt that he had earned Lisa's respect and approval. They both shared many tears, hugs and undying love for each other, and this will be etched in my mind forever.

Ava, a Time to Reflect

27/08/2016

I write this with tears in my eyes, love in my heart and fear in my soul. Dearest Ava, what an amazing impact you've had on our lives. For me you have replaced a glass of wine after a long, hard day. Ava, you are my happy place. You take me to so many wonderful places when we play, and your love for me is unconditional. You look at me through innocent eyes and see things in me that no-one else ever would.

> Ava, you are my happy place.

Tonight, we were talking about scan results and didn't even realise Ava was listening. Once again she asked, "Are you still sick, Lisa?" She's been asking this question a lot lately. "Are you all better, Lisa?" Such innocence in her voice when she asks me these questions, innocence in her face, innocence in her heart, I sometimes wonder if she knows. I mean really knows. Does she know that one day Aunty Lisa won't be there to play Supergirl and Spiderman? That one day we won't be able to retreat to our secret hideout together and dance to our own beat in front of the mirror? I won't be there to be her best friend for the day because, as we all know, these kids are fickle as fuck. One day I'm her BFF and the next day it's Nanna. But one day I won't even be in the running, do you know that, Ava?

Ava you will be three on Sunday, a day I never in my wildest dreams thought I would be here for but had always hoped I would be. I've always said I want to see her go to 'big school' (kindergarten in Australia). I want to be there at her first day of school, watching her get excited weeks before school starts and wanting to try on her uniform and model it for me, showing me her new school bag, lunch box, and pencil case filled with pencils that will create amazing stories of monsters and princesses and drawings of Mum, Dad and her puppy Trixie. Oh, I can only imagine what those pencils will create. I want to stick one of her creations on my fridge and show her amazingness off to everyone who graces my kitchen.

Ava, you're the closest thing to a cure for cancer that I've come across. You pick us up when we're falling into the cancerous chasm. You have this innate sense that I've never seen in any other child, but I'm probably a little biased. All you have to do is look into my eyes or hear a different tone in my voice and you know I'm not well today. You have a warm and caring heart that reaches far beyond any other human being I've ever known.

Ava, you are a star that shines that little brighter than all the others. You were brought into this world eight days before I found out my cancer was back and that I was dying. You've never known any different; you've only ever known sick Lisa.

I want you to know that sick Lisa has tried her best to be as active an aunty as possible, even with her limitations. The healthy Lisa would have climbed that tree with you. She would have picked you up and flown you around the room with your arms outstretched like the superhero you are. She would have wrestled. Boy, would she have wrestled. She would have rolled around on the floor for hours, putting you in pretend choke holds and letting you beat her. Healthy Lisa would have done so many fun things with you, the type of things that mums and dads don't want you to do. But for now you have sick Lisa, and believe me Ava, sick Lisa tries so hard to pretend to be healthy Lisa.

Those secret times that I do pick you up, when the pick-up patrol isn't watching, they hurt. I try not to let you see that when I'm carrying a pretend injured Ava to a pretend ambulance, my tumours are pulling and stretching with every step. I try and hide that from you. It's not just because I don't want you to miss out, it's because I don't want to miss out also. While other people are giving you pretend horsy rides on their back, I'm watching, and with every fake gallop and pretend neigh, my heart is breaking inside knowing that I can't just get on the floor and horse around with you also.

Ava, we've been given so much more than we ever thought we would get. But we've also had so much stolen from us. This cancer cloud that hangs over us every day, threatening to rain on our parade, is so unfair. Every night when you give me my kiss and hug goodbye, I can't help but think, *Will this be the last? The last kiss, the last hug, the last time we sing the wrong words to* Let it Go *together?*

I am sick, Ava. I am really sick. But for some reason, some higher power is keeping me around, keeping me in pain, keeping me in fear and keeping me in your arms. Ava, all the bad stuff — all the pain and suffering — is worth it if I can continue to be bossed around by you and maybe be the chosen one today. The one you call your best friend.

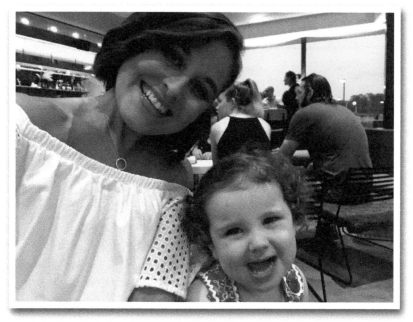

16 December 2015
A family tradition — Lisa and Ava spending a relaxing afternoon at Orion Hotel, Springfield Central, after having family Santa photos taken.

Ava and Lisa shared a special kind of love. Lisa could be having the worst day, but the moment Ava walked into the room a smile would cross her face and she would find the energy to have fun with her. It could be something as little as covering each other with make-up, or on a good day making up a silly dance and putting on a show for the rest of us. There was no-one that could compare to Ava as far as Lisa was concerned.

I often thank God that Ava was born into this situation, that she didn't have to know the heartbreak of getting used to it like we did. Ava knew if Lisa was well enough she would play with her and have fun. But she also knew that when Lisa was unwell, it wasn't Lisa's fault and they'd make up for it when she was feeling better. Ava was a child with an adult head at times. Not only was she Lisa's reason for living, she was also the family's reason for living. She still is.

"Joie de vivre."

Dream Holiday and Nightmare Pain

21/09/2016

The trip of a lifetime: warm turquoise waters of the Indian Ocean lined with red cliffs and pure white sands. The view alone from the aeroplane would have been enough for me to have felt that my dream was being fulfilled. But luckily for my parents and I, the plane landed in Broome. We were welcomed by the warm evening air and the warm heart of a Fabulous Rockstar who had left a wheelchair from her pharmacy in our apartment along with a basket filled with all the necessities one would need when arriving late to a sleepy beachside town.

The photos are beautiful, as are the memories. No-one looking from the outside in would ever be able to tell the fear and pain that lie behind our holiday grins. I'm not saying that we didn't enjoy the trip, far from it. We enjoyed every minute, from floating in the warm waters of Cable Beach to walking through a caravan park in Roebuck Bay to Town Beach and saying to my dad, "Did you hear that sound coming from the grass?" It sounded like something big was slithering beneath and I certainly wasn't going to be rummaging through the weeds to find out what it was.

We walked over the beautiful red rocks and collected shells for my mum's next soon-to-be-started-but-never-completed craftwork for Ava. Dad and I got to Town Beach and upon our return, we noticed a sign in front of where we had previously walked and heard the slithering: 'Do not enter. Reptile breeding habitat'. Oops, well, we had to get back to the car. So with thongs (or flip flops – whatever you like to call them) on our feet, we braved the walk back. Yeah, you read it right. We braved a horny snake pit the other day. Now I don't know about you, but I'm pretty sure a snake getting lucky wouldn't appreciate being interrupted mid-root in the grass. But we made it through to the other side unscathed.

Crazy snake orgies aside, we spent hours lazing on the beach, reading magazines and books – things that you never get the time to do when you're at home. We visited Chinatown, which is basically Broome's town centre, went and had a look at the charming outdoor cinema, strolled through Johnny Chi Lane, visited the Taste of Broome that showcases the local musical and film-making talent and ate the satay skewers that are a Broome breakfast staple. It's actually called the Broome Breakfast. Satay chicken for breakfast – count me in and don't skimp on the rice!

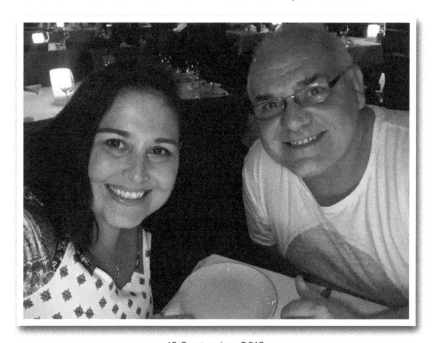

16 September 2016
Lisa and her dad Peter at dinner, enjoying the breathtaking sunsets of Broome, WA. We knew what lay ahead of us but could pretend for now.

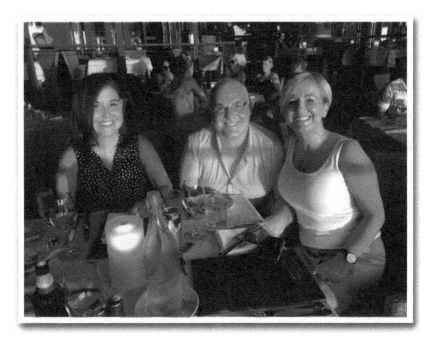

18 September 2016
Sunset dinner at Cable Beach, Broome.

And oh the sunsets. OMFG THE SUNSETS!!!!!

Sitting sipping on a glass of champagne at the Sunset Bar and Grill right opposite Cable Beach, watching the sun descending into the horizon and slowly dipping its feet in the azure waters of the Indian Ocean. When you don't think it could get much better than this, once the sun has completely disappeared into the ocean, the burning oranges and raging reds envelop the sky with grey clouds floating above. The next thing to overpower the senses is the line of camels that are escorted along the beach. In fact, if I'm really honest and not being all poetic about it, the smell of the camels hits you in the face way before the camels come into sight. But still, an amazing sight all the same. (The smell is not so great though; let's just say it lingers a little.)

As I sit here reminiscing about our dream come true, the reality is I'm in so much pain. My liver tumour has not let up since Sunday evening. I'm glad the bastard gave us three full days of just average pain, but shit am I paying for it now. I cannot take in a full breath. The last time I looked at the clock last night was actually 5.30 this morning. I was waking every 20 minutes or so to this indescribable pain radiating from my lower right abdomen to my lower back. Nothing I can do, no position I can lie in, no pain meds I can take, no increase in the dreaded dexamethasone – the drug I've called the devil's drug before. Nothing I seem to have done in the last few days has even nibbled at my pain levels, and they just keep hanging around. Not bad enough that I'd take up a bed in A&E and not weak enough to be able to just ignore it. It's a frigging horrible pain, not unbearable but not quite bearable. What do you do when you're in this position?

I have radiation on Thursday, so I just keep thinking, *Please, hold off. If you're a slow bleed or if you're necrosis or another tumour has popped, please just be bad pain that I can put up with until Thursday.* I'm heartbroken and frightened. I know you Fabulous Rockstars have a decent idea of what our daily struggle is like, but as honest as I am about it, I don't tell you every time I have an ache or a pain. If I did, I would be forever writing about it, and who really wants to read about that shit all the time? No-one. So I really only write about it when I feel it's relevant, and tonight it's relevant.

I know I've made it pretty much three years longer than any specialist thought I would upon initial diagnosis of my metastatic gastric/pelvic sarcoma cancer. But we haven't made it this far drinking wine and staring at sunsets. Those days are fabulous, but the days in between those are not always so fabulous with the chemo, immunotherapies, radiation, surgeries, countless emergency department visits and hospital stays.

Some days I hobble around the house like a woman with arthritic knees. I regurgitate everything I eat or drink. I'm so nauseated that I crouch in the foetal position and my body spasms and cramps into a twisted pretzel. I haven't driven my own car in months because I fall asleep from the pain meds every few minutes. I can't play with my niece on the floor or pick her up when her head and the wall have had a fight and the wall has come out on top.

I fall asleep on the toilet after waiting 20 minutes at a time trying to squeeze a pee out of a bladder that has a couple of golf-ball-sized tumours acting as road blocks to my imprisoned piss, only to be gifted in the end with a stop-

and-start dribble. The many tumour bleeds I've had are all possibly fatal, but the worst pain of all is the 'unknown' – the one that hangs around for days and just won't let up. I can barely sit, barely walk, barely breathe, and every simple movement is planned in my head beforehand with military precision. The simple act of getting up out of your seat becomes an expedition, which takes so long it sometimes feels like it requires food provisions. And mental anguish ... well, let's write a whole other blog on that one another day!

Today is one of those days. With every hit of pain I push the lump in my throat further down, occasionally feeling an escapee tear rolling down my cheek. I'm afraid of that unknown factor:

What if I fall asleep tonight and I bleed out?
What if I collapse in pain and can't get to hospital in time to treat it?
What if I accidentally overdose from giving myself too many pain meds?

Even though I'm sitting here in what most would class as 10/10 pain, I'm still convincing my pain that it doesn't need an ambulance. We don't need to rush to the hospital. I'll just sit here and write about it instead, hanging onto a hope and a prayer that the pain will dissipate overnight. I can reminisce about my dream trip to Broome again without tumour pain muddying the turquoise blue waters of my mind.

I'm sure I will get lots of blog mileage out of this holiday. Pain or no pain, the last few days have been beyond perfection. It will forever remain at the forefront of our minds as one of the most kick-arse experiences of our lives, all thanks to the generosity of an amazing charity, Dreams2Live4.

> Pain feels better
> when you've
> got a tan.

Here I am, sun-kissed, relaxed and in pain. But just like we all think we look better with a tan, it's the same with pain. Pain feels better when you've got a tan.

For anyone that has ever been to Broome in Western Australia, you will know it is one of the most beautiful places on earth. The beaches and sunsets are just out of this world. Lisa, Peter and I were kindly donated this holiday from Dreams2Live4. They are a beautiful charity that does amazing work making dreams come true for those that suffer from metastasised cancer.

In a lot of ways, the trip couldn't have come at a better time. We were stressed, we were tired, and we were frightened. Living in our home felt like sitting on a ticking time bomb 24/7. Yes, we'd be bringing that ticking time bomb with us, but the change of scenery would do us all good. Lisa had talked often of seeing Broome, and we were thrilled that she was going to get the opportunity.

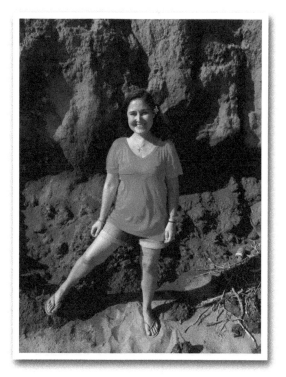

17 September 2016
Lisa at Red Dirt Cliff, Broome. Lisa was so happy to make this trip. Dreams2Live4 made it all possible and we are eternally grateful.

As always travelling was our biggest concern. What if Lisa had a bleed in the air? What if she took a blockage whilst we were away? The hospital in Broome was a small country hospital and wouldn't have the equipment nor the expertise to look after Lisa. But when all was said and done it was Lisa's decision, and for all my worries and fears, I absolutely agreed we should go.

It was evident that Lisa's health was deteriorating fast, and if we didn't take calculated risks now, there wouldn't be a second chance. The palliative nurses gave us a crash course in refilling the pain driver and administering pain meds. Although they were anxious that we were going so far away, they too knew that Lisa's opportunities to experience life were fast coming to an end. It was now or never.

201

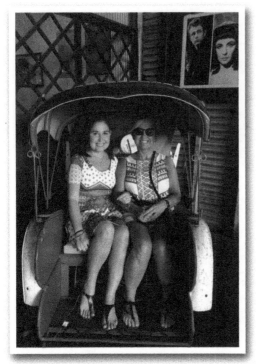

16 September 2016
Lisa and Geraldine at the open-
air cinema in Broome.

As bad as the pain became by the end of the trip, I have to say Lisa was the happiest I had seen her in a long time. The beauty of Broome and relaxed atmosphere were so therapeutic. Although our problems still existed, they were pushed to the back of our minds and we just enjoyed being together in the most beautiful surroundings. We knew that we would be back to reality with a thump in a few days, but for now we savoured the peace and tranquillity whilst recharging our batteries for what lay ahead. This was definitely special, quality time, which we would never forget.

All Hail Kale

24/09/2016

My name is Lisa and I am a lazy cancer patient. There I said it! I can finally breathe. I feel like a tonne of weight has been lifted off my shoulders.

I am that person who receives an email, looks at the subject line and when it says 'Corn – the New Answer to Cancer' I trash it! I'm sorry!!!! I know you've taken the time out of your busy day to think about me and that's so beautifully kind of you. But it's just not me.

I'm not that girl who will drink her own urine that's been heated to 38.5 degrees Celsius, mixed with turmeric and blended with gold dust. I am a lazy cancer patient. I have NEVER tried anything that isn't a prescribed treatment by a medical professional other than one thing, which for the sake of this blog we will call 'oregano'. (Note: It wasn't oregano.)

I was in the worst position I had been in throughout my entire disease. I had been overdosed on pain meds by paramedics and rendered unconscious. Upon return to the world of the living, my left foot had stopped working, and due to my two golf-ball-sized tumours in my bladder pressing on a nerve, my bladder had stopped working. I'd had two consecutive tumour bleeds, blood transfusions and radiotherapy. I was in immense pain, nauseous and desperate.

My dad especially was deeply affected by my pain. He couldn't bear seeing me curled up in the foetal position, tears rolling down my face, moaning and groaning uncontrollably. So he did some research and presented me with the 'oregano' option. I took the prescribed dose, which is less prescribed and more 'anecdotal'. I took one smidgen of the 'oregano', dropped it under my tongue, then mixed the rest with some juice and drank it. The problem with this is a 90-kilogram man would be having the same dosage as myself, and I was only 38 kilograms at the time.

Moments after the first consumption of my 'oregano' I was losing it. My head was spinning, and I was nauseous. I was so paranoid, I demanded that someone be in the room with me at all times because I felt like throwing myself off the balcony. I ate like a horse, and I just remember thinking to myself that I will never be 'normal' again. I thought this 'oregano' had caused me permanent mental health issues. Thankfully, it eventually left my system, after a good ten hours mind you! I am totally supportive of using 'oregano' as a pain relief option and a possible cure to cancer. I just need it to be regulated so that I'm never going to experience an overdose again.

Again, I completely respect those that try alternative treatments. In fact, I envy your self-control. I'm of the school where I think to myself, *Well, things really couldn't get much worse, so stuff it. I'll drink that champagne and eat that bag of corn chips.* I simply don't have the will power, the energy or the commitment to be trying every new fad.

If I was to try every suggestion that my beautiful friends have so lovingly investigated for me, I would NEVER have the time to scratch my arse. I'd be too busy smearing manuka honey on it!

Kale is the new wonder drug. Turmeric is the new wonder drug. Juicing is the new wonder drug. Cut out sugar, gluten, lactose, fructose … basically anything that resembles something edible. Cut it out RIGHT NOW! Do yoga in the morning facing due north whilst humming Hanson's *MmmBop* and wearing no underwear. Brush your teeth anti-clockwise while standing on one foot burping the national anthem, and for God's sake double knot your shoe laces. Ain't nobody got time for rogue shoe laces when you're walking ten kilometres backwards every waning gibbous moon because all of these things will in fact kill cancer.

We cancer patients can also be compared to a pregnant woman. You know how it becomes perfectly okay to walk up to a complete stranger, rub their pregnant belly and proceed to tell your story of your pregnancy and query the beautiful pregnant Goddess about their labour plan? Well, being a cancer patient is pretty much like that. I got a tap on the shoulder in the ladies toilet queue at the Hugh Jackman concert by a Complete Stranger. "Umm excuse me, but I couldn't help but notice that you have a pain driver. Do you have cancer or something?"

Me: "Yes, I do",

CS: "Oh that's terrible. What kind is it?"

ME: "It's blah blah blah terminal gastric sarcoma."

CS: "Wow, have you tried the raw food diet? My friend had stage 2 breast cancer. She opted out of chemo and started the diet. Within six months there was no sign of cancer. Here, let me give you the number of my raw diet vegan sponsor and they'll happily give you a diet plan that will attack and kill your cancer cells. Oh and are you religious? I'm part of a travelling prayer group. We come to people's houses and cleanse them and their house of all illness."

Thank God the engaged sign clicked over to vacant on a cubicle. That woman was taking the longest shit in the history of shits. I envy her and her shitting prowess. I sit on the toilet … (Oh yeah, you read it right. Gone are the shaky knees of the ominous public toilet squat. I now SIT on the toilet. No toilet paper laid on the seat, no disinfecting it with my hand sanitiser. I take a seat and enjoy the splendour that is a comfortable pee. Do you know how freeing and empowering sitting on a public toilet is? It's amazing. No more hovering precariously over the toilet seat that is always inevitably too high for my vertically challenged self, trying to direct my pee in the right direction because women are not designed to stand up while peeing. So now that I have terminal cancer, I am a Public Toilet Rebel. I take a seat, anywhere anytime, except those aluminium public toilets at the beach; a girl has her limits.) ...

I stand up, flush, and as I'm about to walk out of the toilet, a card with the vegan sponsor's details are slid under the door. Needless to say I didn't start the raw food diet. Thankfully, by some divine intervention, whether it be supporters' prayer, chanting, meditations or my diet, radiation or other treatments, whatever I'm doing I must be doing something right. Three years later and I'm still here, albeit full of abdominal/pelvic tumours and living a new norm of constant drug feeds and micro-sleeps. But I'm still here to type this blog and bitch about New Age hipster coffee enemas that are the next big thing when it comes to cancer treatment.

I am always grateful for wonderful people taking the time out of their day to suggest random things I should try. But please don't be insulted if I, or your friend that you're lovingly encouraging to become vegan, don't take your advice and choose our own path. We just have to do this 'our' way. I couldn't count the times that a friend, stranger or loved one has suggested some form of miracle treatment, and I then feel guilty for not proceeding with it. We love you and we appreciate you, but please understand that we have enough on our plate already without adding steamed aloe vera to it because of its healing enzymes!

In the meantime, Fabulous Rockstars, eat, drink and be merry. And don't forget the optimal healing temperature of your urine drink is 38.5 degrees Celsius. You've gotta be precise with that shit, I mean piss. You know what I mean.

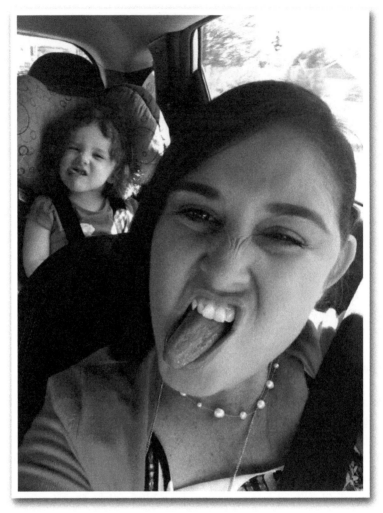

24 September 2016
Lisa and Ava
"All hail kale, all bow downward dog and all will be cured.... Kale? Yuck!" – Lisa

During the early stages of Lisa's diagnosis, I have to admit to being one of those people that believed everything I read and would try my best to convert Lisa. The first attempt was with juicing. I bought the juicer and ingredients, and we got started. But as time when by and the results were continuing to show tumour growth, we both soon lost heart. When Peter came up with the 'oregano' and recommended it to Lisa, we all had high hopes, if not for a cure then at least for pain control. Unfortunately, due to the first bad experience Lisa was resistant to attempt it again until the last few weeks of life. By that stage the disease was too far gone Nothing was going to help.

As any mother would tell you who's going through this nightmare journey, we spend our time on Google looking for that miracle answer. Originally, I would discuss my findings with Lisa. However, it became evident that she wanted me to leave her to her own methods. It was bad enough she was hearing from everyone else never mind hearing it from me at home.

It was strange. I felt bad if I suggested something and Lisa got cranky, and I felt bad if I wasn't suggesting things to make her better too. That's what mums are supposed to do. Truth be told, by the final six months of Lisa's life, I didn't have the energy nor the brain capacity to continue to seek the hidden cure. I could barely get the daily doses of medication right never mind cook up a magic potion I had read about. My head was clogged with dark thoughts and my heart was breaking. I would read Lisa's blogs and wonder how in God's name she found the ability to use humour. All I had to offer was a glued-on smile that I am sure was as transparent as a pane of glass, and I even struggled with that.

By this stage I had become like a new parent, anxiously waiting on Peter to come home from work so I could pass over the baby. Except it wasn't a baby; it was our gorgeous 34-year-old daughter who was dying of cancer. By 7 o'clock I had to take myself off to my room as if I was going to bed, but I wasn't. I was going to my room to mentally refuel. I needed space to try and find the strength to go through it all again the following day. And yes, I felt heart-wrenching guilt: guilt because I needed space, guilt because I was struggling watching Lisa's suffering day in day out, guilt because some days I just wanted to jump on a plane and go hide where I couldn't be found. But most of all I felt guilty because I knew I wasn't coping mentally. I had a daughter dying with cancer, and yet I was the one falling apart. I will never know how Peter coped with all that was going on. He says his work was his sanity, and looking back now, I can fully understand that.

It was around this time that I started going to a counsellor up at the local hospice. I think I did nothing but cry for the first three or four meetings.

> Needing help
> is nothing to be
> ashamed of.

But over time I managed to string a sentence together, and after a month or two I would talk from the minute I went in until the time I left. She was absolutely beautiful. She got me through many of my darkest days and helped me reduce the level of guilt I constantly felt.

Needing help is nothing to be ashamed of. My only regret was leaving it so long.

To Post or Not to Post

12/10/2016

Euthanasia. Just saying the word, or writing it in this case, is often seen as controversial. It's the debate as old as time: Should we be allowed to choose whether to live or die? I realise this blog could lose me some of you Fabulous Rockstars. But please know that this is only an opinion. To be honest my thoughts on this topic have changed regularly from supporting it to not supporting it, just as often as I dye my hair.

I watched a piece on TV on Sunday evening and I felt compelled to finally allow myself to post about it. I've felt it is simply too polarising to write about or too confronting, and I haven't wanted to insult or upset people. I have had a blog about euthanasia sitting for months in my notes. Every now and then I add or take opinions out. Each time I hear it begging for me to copy, paste and post, and each time as I 'Select All' and 'Copy', I end up hitting 'Close'.

The euthanasia debate is like the legalising of drugs debate or the legalising of gay marriage debate. It's usually pulled out by some politician that's trying to distract the public from something else going on, which they don't want you to notice. So hey, let's bring up the euthanasia debate again. That'll distract them!

There will be a vote later on this month in relation to the cross-party Private Members Bill, deciding whether the Voluntary Euthanasia Bill will be debated in the South Australian Parliament. There's something a little different about it this time. This time there has been a campaign with a real human being featured, putting a face to the pain and suffering. Kylie Monaghan, like myself, has spent much of the last few years struggling to live, struggling to fight, struggling to beat cancer. Sadly, Kylie passed away on Saturday. So she will never get to see whether the campaign led to a debate that could potentially change the landscape of terminal illness and the right to die with dignity – the legacy she so greatly wanted to leave for people like me.

Like Kylie I understand why people want the right to choose whether to live or die, and like Kylie I am willing to fight right up until my last breath. I can't ever imagine myself having the strength to say I'm ready to go, never mind voluntarily euthanising myself. But until you've heard the words 'There's no more we can do', until you've fought so hard through the deepest pits of pain, sickness and mental and physical exhaustion or watched a loved one do so, the truth is, you really don't have the necessary pre-requisites to make the decision for thousands of dying human beings. But sadly that is the way of the world. Major life-changing decisions are made by only some chosen few, whilst the rest of us just have to swallow their decision.

> I can't ever imagine myself having the strength to say I'm ready to go, never mind voluntarily euthanising myself.

I realise that people fear that legalising euthanasia, like legalising marijuana for medicinal purposes, would open Pandora's Box, leaving it open to being abused or misappropriated. But with the right legislation and restrictions in place, you shouldn't be able to abuse it.

According to Palliative Care Australia, four per cent of palliative patients' pain cannot be eased or relieved. Not all pain can be alleviated; believe me I know. I am on a pain driver 24 hours a day and still need added pain relief, morning and night in tablet form, as well as injecting pain relief throughout the day. Despite having enough drugs going through my system to make a Colombian drug lord jealous, I still have pain, all day, every day. Granted it's managed pain but pain all the same. It's still there, and if I didn't have this pain plan in place through my palliative doctor, I simply would not be able to function, breathe, walk, talk, you name it.

I've been at the point where I was in so much pain that the doctor took Mum aside and told her that since the amount of morphine I was being given was still not helping my pain, I would simply die from palliative sedation. This is the current practice for palliative care in Australia. Now I may not remember everything about that night, as I was as high as a kite, but I do remember the unrelenting pain, losing the use of my left leg and bladder, and rolling around in a hospital bed moaning. I know first-hand that palliative sedation simply does not cut it. It can take days/weeks for a person to finally die this way, and the entire time their pain is right there with them. I know. I was drugged to the point that a man with the girth of Santa Claus would be rendered dead and still the pain was there, along with the 'pain relief' induced nausea. So in between slowly dying, in pain that cannot be eased, you are also vomiting endlessly, to the point you have nothing left to bring up. You're not eating and you're probably not getting many fluids, other than the IV if they're still running the IV fluids.

Palliative sedation is basically giving a patient morphine over a period of time until the person's body simply shuts down and they die. As I said, doctors and nurses so often say about a patient's death that they died peacefully and in little to no pain. As you all know I love my doctors and nurses. I believe they have one of the hardest jobs in the world, but how do they know that person is not in pain? Just because the patient is so drugged and drowsy and continuously dropping in and out of consciousness does not mean they are not feeling pain. They may well not be, but I know from my own experience that although I was dropping in and out of consciousness, I was still in horrendous pain. It's just that I could no longer communicate to the nurses and doctors that I was.

So is this really a kind way to let a person die? I say no. I say it is a cruel and long, drawn-out process that involves human beings being drugged to the point of numbness. They eventually stop eating and drinking, and we sit and wait. As mentioned before, it could take days or weeks; everybody is different. Do we really want our loved ones to be suffering in such a way after what they've already endured throughout this bastard of a disease? Why would we want them to suffer any more than they have to when there is something we can do about it?

The truth is, restricted drugs like morphine or OxyContin are availed to people in my position very easily. We could, if we wanted to, take ourselves out at any time. I'm sure it's happened time and time again. We would just like to be able to do it legally and without the stigma attached to it. A person gets to the point where they can no longer handle their child, parent, husband or friend having to wipe their arse for them, wash them and feed them. They don't want to drag it out any longer. Have you ever watched a person you love slowly die? Have you ever witnessed a person in your life go from a lively and spirited person to a shadow of themselves that no longer has the desire or the will to live? It is not a pleasant sight for the patient or the loved one. It is literally hell on earth. We don't watch a dog or horse go through untreatable pain and just let nature take its course. We 'put them to sleep'. So why is an animal afforded the option (okay, it's the owner that makes the decision, but you know what I mean) and human beings are not?

I don't often, and may never have, bring up my religion. (I can't actually remember.) In my opinion, your religion is your business and your beliefs are your beliefs. I'm not here to judge you. I believe we should respect each other's beliefs. In my religion, something like euthanasia would be seen as a sin, just as abortion and same sex relationships would be. But I truly believe that we should have the right to choose to die with dignity and in as minimal pain as possible.

> We should have the right to choose to die with dignity and in minimal pain.

I followed a story of a woman who moved to another state in the USA simply so she could be afforded the right to choose when to die. This lady was suffering from debilitating seizures from her brain cancer. She would literally bite parts of her tongue off, and with each seizure came more brain damage, which would impair her ability to communicate. Imagine having these violent seizures. Imagine watching your loved one going through that. Eventually, the young woman decided on a date and she had her nearest and dearest around her bedside. As she took the euthanasia meds over a short period of time, they went around each person in the bedroom and spoke of their favourite stories about her, and she did the same in return. Her husband said that although painful, she went out on her own conditions. No major seizure that took her out. No more pain. She died on her own terms. Doesn't that sound a lot nicer than a palliative sedation?

I hope this blog is taken the way it was intended – an opinion from a person who stares death in the eye every day I wake up. As previously mentioned, I don't believe I could do it myself, but I would never say never. I don't know if my body or my mind for that matter could cope with another bout of untreatable pain. Your body and your spirit can only take so much. I just don't know if I could ever have the strength to legally and voluntarily take my own life. But I believe the option should be out there.

I do not like the idea, much like the medical marijuana situation, of self-administering drugs that have not been properly prescribed. I know there are poor families out there that risk being arrested because they are buying marijuana oil for their epileptic three-year-old child, as it's the only thing that reduces or even eradicates their child's violent seizures. My problem with this is that it has not been properly prescribed, so dosage could be wrong. And we don't actually know what this oil contains. Yes, they say it's pure and blah blah blah, but until there are proper rules and guidelines in place, how do we know that we are not going to overdose our child or ourselves? Euthanasia is the same. It needs to be legalised and regulated so that we can ensure people die in the correct manner and don't get to the point where they decide to just overdose themselves on their own pain medication.

I know this topic is confronting and scary. But for people like me who have terminally debilitating diseases and face imminent death, why not afford us the decency to choose how and when to die? We've already lost so much.

I was really surprised when Lisa decided to write about euthanasia. The incident that Lisa refers to, where the doctor pulled me to one side, was one of the first occasions we thought we were going to lose Lisa. Her pain was excruciating from a bleed from a tumour, and the medical staff could not get it to stop. All they could do was continue to pump her full of morphine to try and ease her pain. The discussion with the doctor was not about palliative sedation. The doctor was explaining that if he continued to give

Lisa morphine, she would slip away when all they were trying to do was stop the pain.

When I went back to Lisa that night, she asked me if she was going to die. As hard as it was I repeated the discussion I'd had with the doctor. Lisa immediately asked that they stop administering the pain relief, and she somehow managed to fall asleep. We were told that night to gather the family as Lisa wasn't going to make it. The next few days went by in a haze. Lisa was given controlled amounts of pain relief and the decision was made to try radiation for the first time. Thankfully, this is what saved Lisa's life, and she was given the gift of another 54 months.

I remember praying that night that God would just put her out of her pain. She'd been through enough. I just wanted her to be at peace. How much more should someone have to deal with this cruel disease? It was pain like I'd never seen before, and I wanted it over.

Since then we've made many wonderful memories. Lisa has seen some of Ava's milestones, and she got to do and see things she'd never seen nor done before. This is what complicates my feelings on euthanasia. I absolutely understand why people want the choice, and I absolutely believe people should not have to suffer as some currently do. But I'm just not sure how I would have felt if Lisa had been given the choice. In fact, looking back, I think I would have been the person that said enough was enough. But Lisa was never going to say it. This is where complications occur as I was her power of attorney, and I was to make the difficult decisions when Lisa wasn't able to. Thankfully, it never came to this.

Bloating and the Birdcage

14/10/2016

They say you should never look a gift horse in the mouth, or in my case the bloated stomach.

I've been gifted the dream of a lifetime by Emirates to attend their Birdcage Marquee as a guest on Melbourne Cup Day. I have been imagining my attendance at this event since I learnt what the Birdcage was. The picture I had in my head was of me with my pre-cancer gloriously-long, shiny hair swishing side from side with a gorgeous headpiece meticulously perched atop. I was svelte and tanned with my stunning designer dress and heels. I was so stunning that Jennifer Hawkins herself hid behind a posh porta loo so that she didn't have to be compared to my gloriousness in the social section of the papers the following day. So that was my idea.

A few years ago, I was all set to attend the Cup, not as a Birdcage guest but as a corporate guest, and I bought this amazing dress. Unfortunately, I didn't get to attend because of flight cancellations and logistics. This dress has been hanging in my wardrobe ever since, and now that I have finally been given this amazing opportunity ... well, that stunning dress? It is now four times too small for me.

This beautiful picture of me swanning around the Birdcage is not what the reality is going to be. I now have a bullfrog chin/neck rather than my pre-cancer strong jawline with not even the glimpse of a second chin. My hair ... at least I have some. And my biggest issue is my ever-swelling, ever-changing belly. I can put a skirt on in the morning, and by 1pm the skirt will no longer zip up due to steroidal swelling and ascites (tumour fluid). One morning I'll wake up looking like I'm six months' pregnant and the next day I look like I'm only three months' pregnant. So you see the dress issue is an actual issue. Have you ever noticed that any stylish dress that would be suitable for the Cup is either fitted or boned? The chances of finding a stylish dress that allows for a changing body throughout the day are slim. Something I haven't been for a very long time.

I went dress shopping with my mum the other day and it was like our own version of *Freaky Friday*. For years I've traipsed from shop to shop, change room to change room, trying to squeeze Mum into dresses that simply wouldn't go near her. It used to upset me that she had so much trouble finding a dress. Now it's the other way around. I almost need to bring WD40 to get me into dresses in double digits sizing. And NOTHING, and I mean NOTHING, came close to my beautiful Melbourne Cup dress that hangs in my wardrobe, waiting to go to the ball, or in my case the Cup.

At one point I was wrestling with a dress, pulling it over my head and desperately trying to not get my make-up on it. I don't know if it's my hormones or if it's the meds, but I sweat profusely all the time. I could have run a marathon before cancer and not had a drop of sweat escape from my pores. Now it pours out of me if I walk from the lounge room to the kitchen. And no, I don't live in a mansion. So I was wrestling with this straitjacket of a dress and Mum comes to the change room door and asks my opinion of the dress she's wearing. Yep, you guessed it. It's the exact same frigging dress and she looks absolutely stunning. Cue every possible emotion a daughter can feel when their mum looks hotter than they do. I think a bit of The Divinyls' *I'm Jealous* was literally on repeat in my mind.

I realise some of you out there will be thinking that you can't please this bloody girl. But believe me when I say that I am more than grateful for the generosity of so many of you out there, especially Emirates. I sort of liken it to getting married. For many of you beauties out there, the thought of getting married has been with you since you knew what it was, drawing big meringue dresses with tiaras and 10-foot-long veils, ten-tier cake, oh and maybe throw a groom in the mix as well.

> I used to draw fascinators on the back of my exercise books and run to the library to watch 'The Race that Stops a Nation'.

Well, that's sort of what it's like for me and my love affair with the Birdcage and Melbourne Cup. At school I used to draw fascinators on the back of my exercise books and run to the library to watch 'The Race that Stops a Nation'. Even if it meant missing the first train home after school and hanging around a train station platform for another hour. I would eagerly wait for the evening news download on all the fashions on the field and the newspaper the next day.

So imagine you suddenly balloon, have two or three chins and are so bloated that it is not only painful, it literally takes your breath away (tumours sitting high in my abdomen push on my lungs, literally suffocating me), and your wedding is tomorrow. I'm sure when you were picturing your special big day, you didn't envisage a completely different looking person to yourself. Well, that's what it's like for me. My body and my face change shape and appearance from one day to the next, and it's just sad that I'm not feeling my best physically or emotionally for my special day.

I know I should be screaming in joy from the rooftops, but I'm scared the dress I've bought will not zip up on the day. If it doesn't, I simply cannot go because I literally have nothing else in my wardrobe that is Cup-suitable and stretchy enough to allow for my ever-expanding belly. I've also had the amazing offer from a fabulous milliner to make my head piece on the day, and I'm scared that I'll get his piece and then change my dress at the last minute for comfort reasons.

Anyway, as I've said before, just because I have cancer, just because I am terminal, does not mean my insecurities have just disappeared into thin air. So many people in my position begin to say things like "Appearance doesn't matter" or "There are so many more important things in life like actually living". Well, I'm not one of them. I still have my insecurities and I always will. Right up until the end I'll probably be checking my reflection in the doctor's stethoscope. If you unlock my phone, you'll be greeted by your own face because I'm constantly looking at myself on my camera in my phone.

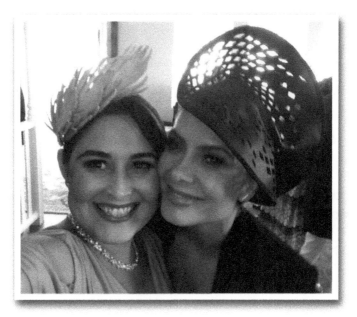

1 November 2016
Lisa and singer Natalie Bassingthwaighte at The Birdcage at the Melbourne Cup. A conversation struck up in the Ladies ended with a drink and a selfie requested by Natalie. Such a gorgeous girl.

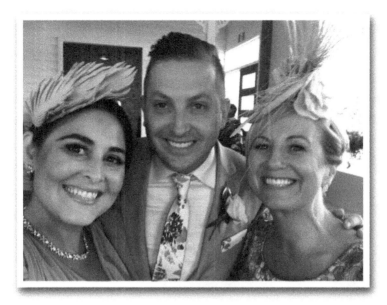

1 November 2016
Lisa, Geraldine and John Caldwell at
The Birdcage, Melbourne Cup. John Caldwell was the amazing guy who made
Lisa's dreams come true. He reached out to Lisa often and was always a
great support to me during the toughest of times. We are eternally grateful.

Whatever happens, I just hope my face and stomach are less bloated that day and I can do my zip up and breathe the whole day. If that happens I will be ecstatic. Thank you, Fabulous Rockstars, for getting me into the magical land of unicorns, WAGS and the 'beautiful' people. Keep your fingers crossed that Megan Gale or Jen Hawkins don't rock up in the same dress as me because that would just open up a whole other can of worms. That I just couldn't deal with on top of everything else. On the upside it would make a good blog!

One of the things our family were truly blessed with whilst Lisa was ill was the kindness of others. Being a family that has always worked for what we had made it extremely difficult for us to ask for help when it was needed. However, when it came to Lisa's bucket list of experiences, we set our pride aside and turned to those determined to support us – the *Terminally Fabulous* followers.

Through the blog we came across a lovely lady called Marla McCauley-Zell. Marla and her son had previously done some charity work with an amazing guy called John Caldwell, who is a media commentator for Channel 10. Marla made one quick call to John explaining Lisa's plight and John immediately kicked into action. Within a week of contacting John, he had the Channel 10 film crew in our lounge and was interviewing Lisa live. Talk

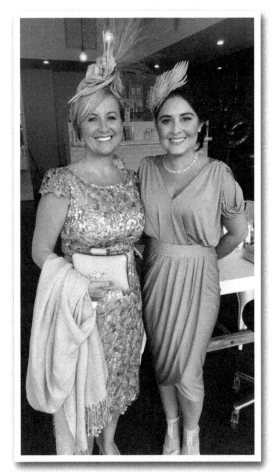

1 November 2016
Geraldine and Lisa ready for the races at The Birdcage, Melbourne Cup. Lisa's gifted dress was perfect, as was the day!

about surreal. Two minutes later a representative of Emirates Airlines walked in and presented Lisa and I with a beautiful gift of entry to the Birdcage, flights and accommodation. We were beyond ecstatic. As part of the gift, Lisa would also receive a dress of her choice from a formal dress store and a bespoke headpiece by the amazing Neil Grigg. We were blown away by such kindness. I have maintained contact with these gorgeous people who I now consider special friends.

I was so excited about the trip as I knew how much it meant to Lisa. But underneath I was feeling anxious. Lisa had been having issues finding clothes that suited her everchanging body shape and were comfortable to wear as tumours were now protruding from her abdomen and pelvis. Fluid had also become a big issue.

We went to the boutique to select a dress, but the styles were too fitted for Lisa. There was one dress that looked beautiful on her, but as much as she liked it I could tell she was disappointed that she could no longer select the tightly-fitted style she once could have worn. She didn't want to seem ungrateful, but there was disappointment written all over her face. When we got home, Lisa tried the dress on to show the family. They thought it was beautiful, but Lisa felt they were being kind.

By the time we got to race day, Lisa had bought another four dresses and had one made just in case. The gifted dress was the dress she wore, and she looked absolutely amazing. Our make-up, hair and transport were donated by other blog followers and we were treated like queens throughout. Experiences like this have changed me and my outlook on life. They have

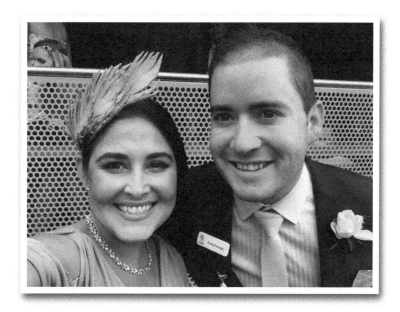

1 November 2016
Lisa and Danny Connolly at The Birdcage, Melbourne Cup. Danny reached out to Lisa on Terminally Fabulous and arranged for Lisa to visit his company's venue and The Birdcage. They remained firm friends until the end and we have continued with that friendship.

made me more determined to work hard to give back to others in difficult situations. I hope to one day set up a charity that will ease the terminal journey for both patients and their carers.

Emergency Department Guilt

07/11/2016

I wrote this blog last week, just a couple of days before I flew down to Melbourne for the trip of a lifetime. But I didn't really want to post it in case people got concerned about me pushing myself to go to the Cup. Believe me, my health comes before any amount of celebrities caged in one area, and I would never put myself at risk just to catch a glimpse of the girls from *The Block*...

So there I was last Sunday in excruciating pain, once again doing the should-I-or-shouldn't-I-go-to-the-hospital argument in my head. I'm in my bedroom in insurmountable pain, the type of pain where every time I attempt to inhale, it feels like my liver is being stabbed by a blunt, rusted knife and my lungs are being suffocated by the sheer size of my tumours. The problem is, I've been in this pain before and it has subsided after an hour. And I've been in this pain before and within hours been told I'm not going to make it through the night due to the amount of blood loss from a tumour bleed. So which one is it? Is it the I'm-going-to-die pain or the It's-going-to-subside pain?

I don't have X-ray glasses that can see into my abdomen and tell me if it's: a tumour bleed; a tumour has popped; tumour necrosis; my bowels that have moved, forcing a tumour to hit a nerve causing pain; tumour growth; constipation; ascites and the list goes on. So it's no wonder I have this back and forth with myself every time I feel pain. Then my poor parents get it as well. I'm usually asking them, "What do you think? Yes or no?" to which they reply, "Only you can tell us that. We can't feel the pain". Then I get annoyed at them because they won't make the decision for me. Then when they say, "We think you should be in hospital," I usually object anyway. The poor bastards can't win.

So on Monday night, I was doing my usual back and forth and then took a few breakthrough pain injections that did nothing. That was it. My little argument in my head wasn't an option. The pain had me in a chokehold and I couldn't tap out. Time to go to emergency. No time to ring the ambulance – just get me there.

In my mind, this time I was dying. At every bump and turn, I was yelping like a neglected dog in pain. Anyone who knows me knows that if hospital can be avoided, I will avoid it at all cost. So this car trip is a good 30-minute ride, and every second I felt like pain was seeping from every pore. If I cry it's more painful and all I wanted to do was bawl. So every now and then crying would start and the pain would rush over me, causing distress in my breathing, which in turn caused even more pain. My poor dad was watching on, helpless while trying to drive the car and holding my hand like I was giving birth. I have a feeling a few red lights were ignored that night and the speedo may have been in overdrive.

Emergency departments are for the most part amazing. My own experience with them is usually 10/10. The triage nurse or admin person at the counter usually sees the pain written all over my face and my contorted body upon arrival and rushes out with a wheelchair or directs us through the hallowed doors that lead to triage. On a few occasions, I've had really difficult experiences. Some hospitals seem to lack a sensitivity chip in their ED front desks. I don't know if it's how they've been trained, so that they don't become emotional or affected by what may appear before them. But one thing's for sure: I've been to EDs all over Australia and there are some I'd prefer to avoid at all costs.

> Some hospitals seem to lack a sensitivity chip in their ED front desks.

No person that approaches an emergency department with a genuine illness or medical issue should be made to feel that they are an annoyance. Do you really think that doubled over in pain in your waiting room is where I imagined my Sunday going? Do you think I'm here just for fun, for a laugh?

You see, I already suffer from ED Inferiority Complex (EDIC). I don't think it's an actual recognised complex, but it's what I call it anyway. I never feel that my pain or illness is worthy of taking up an ED bed, so when I'm faced with an uncaring person at the counter, who tuts when she sees me walking in because she's standing there with her heated bolognese from last night's dinner and would rather be splattering sauce down her chin than take the time to assess my case appropriately, it pisses me off.

I've had an occasion where we've been ambulanced in and people have been nothing but downright rude to us. My brother and his wife rushed to the hospital to see what was going on and the admin lady came out to us in the hall, yelling at my family for taking up waiting room space and to move them! Why not just ask them to go to the café politely? You don't need to publicly shame them for caring for their sister. I've also been forced to sit in a chair even though I kept telling them I couldn't sit. Once I went to the toilet, came back out and found they had given the bed away and left a chair for me to sit on, even though they knew I was physically unable to. On that occasion my mum ended up in tears, and she's a stoic woman. It takes a lot to make her cry, but she just felt that the hospital did nothing but make us feel like a nuisance from the time we arrived. And by the way, it wasn't us who sent us to ED, it was my GP who told us to rush to the hospital even after I begged her to not make me go.

My ED Inferiority Complex is really bad. I always believe that someone else is worse off than me. From the 21-year-old with alcohol poisoning to the ice addict scratching their flesh to the bone, the little girl with a fish hook stuck in her finger to the bloke who was building an IKEA flat pack and obviously didn't follow instructions properly because he now has a piece of MDF attached to his forearm ... and don't even get me started on the woman who came in with lock-jaw ... Let's just say her partner was slightly embarrassed explaining that one to the triage nurse ... I've seen it all and I always feel they should be seen before me.

A wonderful emergency department nurse once told me, after I had told her about my EDIC, that in fact I was probably more important than most in the waiting room. That's because, unlike the fool who thought it was a smart idea to try riding a unicycle on the balcony of a five-storey building, I didn't choose to get cancer and certainly didn't choose to be terminal and have tumour bleeds that require blood transfusions, embolisations and radiation to stop them. She told me that this is out of my hands, so they should be saving me and keeping me around for as long as they can. Whereas I think, because I'm already 'dying', why would you want to waste valuable time and resources on keeping me going, only to remain an ongoing strain on the already struggling health system? It simply doesn't make sense.

She replied, "Do you think the man that we've just treated for falling down the stairs and spraining his ankle isn't a strain on our health system? He's an alcoholic. His disease is and will continue to be a strain on our health system until he either gets irreparable liver damage and dies or decides to get help. Either way his alcoholism will continue to be a strain on public health resources, just like yours does. So why should your life be any less important than the next? We are all human and we all deserve equal and fair access to the public health system." That nurse was so right, and one day, maybe, I'll realise that saving my life is just as important as saving yours.

Remember, A&E is for emergencies not ingrown toenails or runny noses. But if you have a serious health issue, don't suffer from EDIC. Get your sick butt to your local hospital and hopefully you'll be greeted by a fabulous triage like I have been so many times before.

> A shout-out to all you fab triage and ED admin out there!

99.9 per cent of triages are fabulous! A shout-out to all you fab triage and ED admin out there!

One thing our family has always said is that we could not complain about the medical service we have received in Australia. As you can imagine, we feel like experts in hospital protocol. There have only ever been two occasions when we have had a real issue. As the patient or support person you have no idea what else is going on in that department. Yes, you can see they are busy, but you don't know who has to take priority and who doesn't.

Unfortunately, the day I had a minor meltdown it was a Monday and crazy busy. We had waited just over an hour for an ambulance, which is extremely rare, and when we got to the Emergency Department, the ambulance trolleys were queuing out the door. Due to Lisa's pain levels on this day, and the amount of pain medication she had already received without having impact, we feared the worst – a bleeding tumour. Having to queue was extremely difficult as time is critical with a bleed. However, Lisa was taken off a trolley and told to sit on a chair, which she found impossible. I became terribly upset, which was highly unusual for me, but I felt that this situation was diabolical.

Whilst in tears, I asked if I could take Lisa to another hospital as it was obvious that the head nurse wanted the trolleys cleared from where they were lining the hallway. They said that to move her to another hospital where there was no guarantee that she'd be seen any sooner would be irresponsible. So now not only was I upset because of Lisa's pain levels, I felt like I was being shamed into staying where we were. Thankfully, they agreed to put Lisa back on the trolley and a doctor came out into the hallway and could see how upset I was and understood my fear. He scanned Lisa there and then and took her bloods. Within minutes it was confirmed that there was no bleed and we were able to go home.

I think it's fair to say Emergency Departments must see and hear a fair amount of complaints. However, I felt that I was automatically categorised as one of those people that was never happy during this experience. I was in floods of tears. It was a busy day and my priority was Lisa, even if I felt that she wasn't theirs. I think I was also starting to realise that Lisa was deteriorating. Her immune system was weak, every part of her body hurt, and her bowel and bladder were starting to block more frequently.

I was scared.

I'm Not Ready to Be a Fading Memory...

10/11/2016

I've spoken before about a moment I had standing at the kitchen bench looking over our loungeroom and watching my mum, dad, brother Steven, Marianne my sister-in-law and Ava, my then two-year old niece. They were just going about a normal night, sitting and chatting, laughing at Ava while the TV was on in the background, unnoticed. In that moment, I realised that one day that will be their new normal – going about life without me in it.

They won't be thinking of me or calling out to me to put the kettle on while I'm in the kitchen. I will be the metaphorical TV: there but not really.

There will be times like birthdays and Christmases when I will be remembered, when they'll talk about how I was the hardest person to buy for when it came to presents. As much as they think it's because I just can't be pleased, I think it's more to do with the fact that I've never learned to accept gifts graciously. I'm not a good receiver because I never feel deserving of the gift. A great giver, yes. There's just always been something that doesn't sit right with me when receiving a gift, like I'm unworthy of it or their money could be spent on something more important. I've had to learn over recent months, especially, to receive gifts better. I've been gifted some beautiful gifts from some Fabulous Rockstars, like my dream trip to Broome by Dreams2live4 and the trip to the Melbourne Cup by Emirates. So I've had to receive some pretty bloody big gifts of late.

I've learnt that to be able to give, you must be able to receive. That wonderful, warm feeling that comes over me when I see the happiness on a person's face upon receiving my gift should be experienced by everyone at some point in their life. If I don't allow people to give, I am depriving them of the best gift of all – that warm, fuzzy feeling and moment of pure gratefulness and joy when a person sees a gift for the first time. Gifts don't have to be physical, expensive or huge. Just smiling at the lonely man on a park bench is a gift, for that may be the only human interaction that person has all day, all week. I suppose giving would be my favourite pastime. By writing this blog I'm giving myself to you, and I feel this is the greatest gift I've ever given.

This will be my legacy. When I'm long-gone and nobody remembers the girl who guilted her way into the Melbourne Cup, and *Terminally Fabulous* is just a couple of words that no longer resonate with people, it will still be there for my family, my friends, my loved ones and maybe the odd Google searcher to look back on when they need a virtual hug. This has been my greatest gift so far. I don't think there's much more a person could give of themselves than their complete truth. To bare one's soul publicly has been a gift for me also. I have gained so much joy from Fabulous Rockstars that write and tell me stories of how my blog has helped them or their loved one get through the day. There is no way to describe the feeling you get when you open an email from a complete stranger and they bare their soul to you in return. How amazing is that? People actually feel safe enough disclosing their deepest and darkest thoughts and feelings to me. Yes, with this gift comes sadness, stories of death and devastation, but that warm, fuzzy feeling I get from the good email helps to take the sting away from the sadness.

There will be times when my friends will laugh at the stupid things I've said or done over the years. When the tears from laughter dry on their cheeks, I will be returned to that little drawer in the back of their mind, waiting to be stumbled across again accidentally when looking for something else.

> I'm not ready to be a fading memory.

I do not want to be a memory. I don't want to be talked about, and I certainly don't want to be forgotten. I want to be given a gift that to most sane people is seemingly unachievable. I want the gift of life, the gift of a cure, a miracle. I'm not ready to be a fading memory.

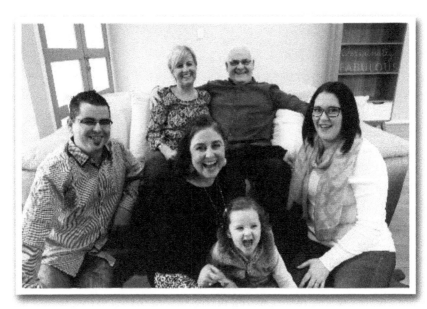

23 June 2016
Steven, Geraldine, Lisa, Peter, Ava and Marianne.

Reading this blog again tells me that Lisa and I were at the same place psychologically. She too was feeling the end was closing in on her, and she was terrified.

So many times she commented that she wouldn't see Christmas, and I would reassure her that she would. But truth be told, I didn't think she would. If it wasn't for the steroids and the bloating she would have been skin and bone. Food wasn't staying down, and the number of meds she was on were making her either ramble constantly or drop in and out of micro sleeps throughout the day. Getting her to go to hospital when her pain was extreme was nearly impossible.

She didn't want to go in as she was frightened she wouldn't get out.

Once again, I firmly believe that it was the love and the support of the *Terminally Fabulous* followers that kept her going. For once in her life she felt like she was truly achieving something; something she had created was having a positive impact on others. The outpouring of love they gave her was her reward. They trusted her, and she knew it. The honesty that got her in trouble at times in the past had now made her a favourite to people around the world, and she was truly proud. We all were.

Shit-scared

16/11/2016

Here we are once again, back in 'that' place I just don't want to be. Mum asked me a very telling question today. "So, are you still wanting your funeral down in Sydney?" Speaks volumes, doesn't it. There's absolutely nothing wrong with that question either. It's completely reasonable in our current situation, and she knows that I've always wanted my funeral to be 'my' way, not the way of some funeral director in a wide-brimmed hat and a chignon bun from White Lady Funerals.

Today, though, practicality wasn't high on my priority list. Number one was to walk around dazed and confused, wondering why we're back in this place again, the place of death. I mean, wasn't a cure supposed to have been found by now? I've stretched it out to three years. I've given you frigging cancer scientists enough time and frigging donations, so why are we still here? I've been frozen in this unknown state for what feels like forever. Haven't some bloody mice in China had their cancer cured from some sort of trial somewhere in Beijing? You can have a face transplant now, and I read somewhere that some Russian guy has just volunteered to be the first human to trial a whole head transplant, and still we can't manage to kill little lumps that keep popping up inside my body. How does this make sense?

In recent days I've had an episode where I was curled up in pain, with my undies around my ankles, on the toilet floor and banging the wall for my mum or dad to get me an enema to help with a blockage from my kilogram of pelvic tumours pressing on my rectum.

I knew it was coming. I knew it was getting worse again, but it still doesn't prepare you.

It doesn't matter how long you have 'terminal' attached to you, you never just get used to it. I know so many of you write how strong I am, an inspiration. But really, I'm not. I'm as shit-scared as I was that Thursday, September the 5th 2013 in that little ultrasound room when the technician gave me the poor-you-your-cancer's-back' puppy dog eyes.

> I actually wish someone was dying with me.

I said to Mum today (and I almost felt wrong saying it but it's the truth, so here goes) "I actually wish someone was dying with me." I know how horrible that sounds, but for fuck's sake, women can't manage to go to the toilet by themselves on a night out, so why would it be so wrong of me to not want to go out (die) alone? I know it's horrible to wish death on someone else, but it's not like I'm saying to mum to take an overdose of my morphine and come along for the ride. I'm simply saying it would be a comforting thought to know you weren't going to be facing this alone.

I know everyone who has strong faith says that the other side is better than this side. But what if it's nothing? What if I die and that's it? The thought of not going on somewhere else after this is what scares me the most. I know I believe in God and I say I have strong faith. But I'm sorry; until someone goes over to the other side with a GoPro attached to their head and comes back with concrete proof of this so-called 'other side' or 'heaven', I simply can't commit to heaven's existence. The thought of not being reconnected with your loved ones once you die scares the shit out of me. I so desperately want to be so blind in my faith that I believe we will be reunited in years to come. It would give me the comfort I so desperately crave. But my fears just override all of it.

I sometimes wonder if it would be easier if I was in my eighties and my loved ones had already passed away. Maybe then the thought of a Great Gatsby themed welcome party upon my arrival at my new home in the sky would be more likely. Maybe I'd be looking forward to it because the ones I love have already gone.

All these thoughts and considerations are swimming around my head, all day, all night.

I'm roaming around at 2am, in between crying, begging and praying for this to be one big joke and for it to all go away. I'm scared to go to sleep in case I'm not going to wake up. The words 'kilo of tumours' keep whirling around in my head like an annoying fucking mosquito in your bedroom at night.

Please, I'm begging you, just leave me alone. You've had your fun. Now pack your bags and move on! I'm looking down at my bloated, tumour-filled belly and asking why. Why did this happen? I'm imagining tomorrow without me in it. How can everyone else still be here at some point and I won't be? It doesn't make sense. It's just one big mind-fuck on Viagra. It doesn't matter how long you fight this bastard of a disease, you still go to bed thinking you'll wake up tomorrow and everything will have miraculously disappeared. Hope is so pivotal. It keeps you going, but I don't seem to face my reality.

Lisa! You're dying! Accept it and move on already!

I just can't!

I wish I could promise you Fabulous Rockstars that tomorrow will be a better day, that I will be more positive. But I'm not in the habit of making promises I can't keep. I can only hope that tomorrow will come, and if it does that I am more positive about my situation. Thank you all for your love, support, positive vibes and prayers. I hope you can appreciate that I don't know how I will behave in coming days. I may go AWOL for a while, or it could be all things as normal. I just don't know.

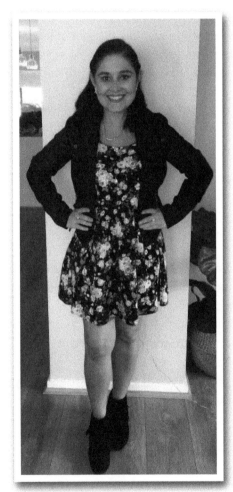

16 November 2016
Lisa

As a mother, these blogs were always the hardest to read. On the one hand, Lisa was wishing she wasn't going to die alone, and on the other I was wishing I could take it from her and it was me not her. But unfortunately, life isn't like that. You get the hand you are dealt, and you have to deal with it as best you can. Truth is, at this stage none of us were dealing with it. It was like being in a room and all four walls were closing in on us, and there was nothing we could do about it. It just wasn't the family that were suffering. All of our closest friends would ring daily, and the desperation was evident when the question was asked, "Well, any change today?"

The answer was always the same or worse. That's the cruel thing about cancer. It can be a long, slow, excruciatingly debilitating journey. Not content enough to make you suffer, it sucks the very life right out of those closest to you. Although we would not be taking the final step with Lisa, we were definitely suffering with her every minute of every day.

Seeing the end getting close, I would have the occasional panic attack, first and foremost about losing Lisa but also about fulfilling her last wishes. If I couldn't take her place in life, I was going to make sure I was clear about her final wishes. And I would do my utmost to make sure they were fulfilled. Where possible I always tried to pick my moment to have these discussions. I'd choose a time when Lisa's pain was under control, when she was happy to talk and when she was also talking openly about her passing, although these times were rare.

As anyone who has been through this journey would know, anger is a common emotion:

> How could God put our baby girl through this?
> Where is our miracle?
> Why is her suffering so relentless, and why do we have to have these discussions?

But when we pushed past these feelings, we realised how much we needed our faith. We had to believe Lisa was going to heaven where she would be welcomed with open arms. We had to believe that she was going to a place that would be filled with so much love and happiness, a place that knew no pain. Otherwise we would have crumbled.

We had to believe Lisa was going to heaven where she would be welcomed with open arms.

Lisa was extremely fond of the local priest where she had lived before moving to Queensland. At this stage, he was more than happy to travel to Brisbane to conduct the funeral mass. So it was decided that we would have the funeral in Queensland.

What's the Returns Policy?

21/11/2016

So here I am nearly a week later. The latest news we've received about my cancer is still just as hard to swallow as a wheatgrass shot laced with pigeon poop. It never gets easier; if anything it gets harder. Oh and did I mention it's 4.30am? No, not an early start. I haven't even slept, what with my increased steroid dosage and the pain from something like 30 tumours in my abdomen and pelvis. Sleeping evades me lately.

> My cancer is still just as hard to swallow as a wheatgrass shot laced with pigeon poop.

I'm still walking around dazed and confused with a constant look plastered on my face that could best be described as something resembling Alicia Silverstone's expression on the *Clueless* DVD cover, except of course, much less blonde, slim and Hollywood C-lister. For those of you wondering what gibberish that all was, I highly suggest you get your Gen Y girlfriends around for a movie night, stat.

The last blog I did, I discussed my fear of death and the unknown afterlife or existence of heaven, even though I consider myself to have strong faith. The thing I admire in people with faith is their unwavering belief that there is something after all of this that is even better than here on earth, and they're not scared of their mortality. I don't know if you can truly know what your feelings about death are until you're faced with it. Before this bastard of a disease, I had no doubt that there was a heaven. But now that I'm faced with my own death, that part of the process isn't so certain.

Sit in a room with your doctor, hear the words, "You have cancer and you only have weeks, maybe months to live," and let's see how at peace you are with it then. I yearn for that peace of mind I used to have. I'm not saying I've lost faith. I'm simply saying my religious GPS hasn't had its recent update. Hopefully, once it has, I will be back on track and comforted by the thought that one day I will be reunited with my loved ones.

Even with the world in the state it's in, here I am trying to figure out how I'm going to keep going, keep breathing, keep moving forward. How am

I going to push through this time? Everyone keeps saying, "You've done it before. You'll do it again". But I've never had this much disease before, and with each radiation the less effective it seems to be. Eventually, it won't work at all. People are so positive that I'll make it, but they're not the ones inside my diseased body. My body has been battling against itself for so long, eventually one

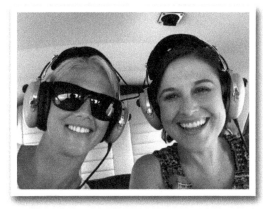

11 January 2016
Lisa and Rebecca Cooper during a girls' trip away at Port Jackson, Sydney, NSW.

of us is going to have to give in. Looking at my recent scans, it seems it's me that's reaching for the white flag.

My days have consisted of constant pain, pain 'relief' (in inverted commas because there is no relief – with every injection my pain remains the same, but the tiredness and confusion momentarily distracts my body from it), lethargy, laxatives, sleeping, and watching enough reality TV and HBO series that I could pick any *True Blood* cast member's arse from a line-up. Probably the worst thing I've done over the last week is to ignore phone calls and text messages.

I've withdrawn from my friends, which I know is wrong. I know they only want to support me, but the sheer energy it takes to make my thoughts connect with my mouth is too much. I love them, they love me, and we hopefully can all remember that. My 'oldest' best friend, my number one in my squad, is Rebecca (or Bec). Rebecca has been by my side through it all, from pimples to palliative care. She's been my rock, and here I am building an emotional wall protecting me from her. I mean, who does that? Who treats their friends like enemies? Me, I do.

As a young terminal cancer patient I often feel guilty for thinking these thoughts. As I sit in my GP's waiting room with my pain driver pumping my life's juice into me, with the word 'palliative' blazoned on the front of it, and the 90-something-year-old woman sits opposite me complaining about her cataract, I can't help but think, *Be grateful you made it. You were one of the lucky ones.* I know it's a truly terrible thought, but it's just that sometimes when life gives you one dried up lemon, it's difficult to hear a person whose had an abundance of fruit baskets complain about it. We simply wish we were that woman. If anything I suppose you could say we envy them. I know it's wrong, but this 'shituation' takes your mind to dark places. I don't hate elderly women. I just wish I was going to get the chance to BE one.

> I'll regret thinking these thoughts and I'll definitely regret publicly posting them.

Thankfully, I read my friend's blog *Dear Melanoma* and she mentioned that she too has the same thoughts. It's one of the reasons she doesn't like to share a room in hospital with elderly women as it's a physical reminder that she's' not going to get to make memories over the next 60 years. Emma, in her mid-20s, is in hospital as a lab rat trialling yet another drug, trying to find something that will either cure her or give her more time. Meanwhile, Betty in bed 320 is buzzing the nurse for the fifth time to complain about the air conditioning. (Betty is a fabrication, purely for editorial purposes. Sadly Emma is not.)

Believe me, in a few days I'll regret thinking these thoughts and I'll definitely regret publicly posting them. But as I always say, I've promised you warts and all, and to start holding back from you now would be wrong.

It's simple. I'm in love with life, and to die is to take away my greatest love.

I hope in coming days that I will be in a better place. I've made contact with my counsellor, so hopefully that will help. I got out of bed today and had a shower, so that's good, and I didn't go back to bed. I actually made it into the loungeroom to watch TV. So whilst myself, my friends and family face the latest plot in our own personal soap opera, I thank you for your love and support. With one radiation down and two more to go, we can only hope and pray that it works. Because quite frankly, if it doesn't I'm fucked.

Stay Fabulous, Rockstars.

The Ups and Downs of Terminal Cancer

30/11/2016

I finally got around to reading some of your messages. Thank you all for your ongoing love and support for a stranger from a little suburb on the outskirts of Brisbane.

One common message I receive lately is that my blogs have become more depressing or sad of late. I suppose you're right, but that's the truth of this disease. You've entered into the world of a 'terminally ill' person not a 'stage-one-99-per cent-cure-rate cancer blog'. It's an incurable cancer blog. Terminal, essentially meaning I am dying. Maybe not today, tomorrow or the day after that, but one day it will take me (unless that miracle happens).

Believe me, it's still as hard for me to say it as it may be for you to read it. It really is a rollercoaster, and the downs just take a little bit longer to ride out. As much as I wish I could be positive Pollyanna all the time, it's impossible to be that.

I promised you a truthful and honest insight into my life. I suppose sometimes I've not been as honest with you as I should have been, especially earlier in my blog. I was new to it and I didn't want to be all death, death, death. There are times that I've blogged and it's all jokes and funny analogies. But they've been more for your benefit than mine. As my blog grew, I received more and more messages from cancer patients and carers, and they were grateful for the truthful parts that so many of us think about – the dirty laundry truth – that we don't want people to know. We feel so guilty for many of our thoughts, like wishing it wasn't us with terminal cancer and that it was someone else or questioning our faith. If we say those thoughts out loud, people may turn against us or be insulted. But that's what I'm here for: to be your voice of reason and truth no matter how hard it may be to swallow.

I have numerous reasons for writing my blog. One is to connect with others including those in our position, so we don't feel so alone. Another is that it's alright to be scared about cancer and dying. You don't have to get to a point that you feel at ease with this disease. Not everybody dies accepting their fate. Another thing I was sick of was the lack of honesty out there about terminal disease: "I do Pilates every day and only eat raw and my cancer is dying" and "This disease makes you enjoy life more." Blah blah blah.

Yes, you may change your diet and ring your mum more, but I don't want to feel guilty because I have terminal cancer and still drink the occasional Coke or eat way more cheese than that food pyramid thing says I should. And as for exercising and meditation, yes, that's good for you. But I can barely reach my arse nowadays to wipe it, never mind attempting a closed leg rocker or bicycle position. Yay for you. I'm all for it if you can do it. I just got sick of reading a blog and by the end of it feeling like I was the son of Lucifer himself for drinking wine. I already have fucking terminal cancer, so don't make me feel bad for going for that fourth slice of pizza or eating burnt toast.

I don't want people to read my blog and feel like they're doing terminal cancer wrong. There is no one way to live when dying. If there was there'd already be a *Dying for Dummies* book out there. Each person that goes through this is a newbie. You can only die once, so no one person is an expert. My advice: Put down the how-to-die-gracefully books and do this terminal disease however the fuck YOU want.

If you want to throw a tantrum and smash a few plates, if you want to swim the English Channel, climb Mt Everest or simply spend your time at home watching every reality show ever made, that's your choice. I never want a person to read one of my blogs and feel like they're doing something wrong. I am no Dalai Lama, certainly not a life coach or psychiatrist, and most importantly I am not God or whoever your higher power is, if you even have one.

> As cancer patients we all too often pretend to be okay for the sake of others.

I've said it before. As cancer patients we all too often pretend to be okay for the sake of others. We want to protect you from the truth because the truth is just way too ugly and scary. A few people have said that they want the upbeat, hopeful Lisa back. Again, I get it. It doesn't upset me that they feel this way. It's because they want to protect their own feelings. If I give up, what do those people, those strangers that care for me or garner hope from me do? How can they be strong if I am weak? I have not given up. I am not resigned to the fact that my cancer has taken me. I'm not about to make that phone call to my cancer and congratulate it on its resounding victory. But the truth of the matter is, this disease will kill me.

I've never changed my thought process in relation to my feelings about my terminal diagnosis. I still hope for the best and prepare for the worst. That little saying was used very heavily in the early stages of my cancer and was definitely my brother Steven's go-to. He'd come into the hospital and say it and leave the hospital saying it.

I love that you beautiful people are concerned for me and worry that I may be giving up. But believe me, if or when I give up, you won't be confused about it. You'll know because I'll tell you. I understand your fear; this is probably pretty new to you. You come across this random blog one day in your newsfeed and you've got a few minutes to spare, so you start to read. And like I have done with other bloggers, you fall into their story; you feel a connection. You feel like you are friends, and you talk about them like you are. We all do it.

My family and I have been dealing with this for years now. So perhaps I can be a little blasé about my health, talking about it like I've got a cold. Many of you Fabulous Rockstars write to me or comment on my blog that you feel we would be best friends if we lived in the same city, state or country. Our connection feels so deep that when I have my down moments and openly blog about them, you feel like you're on the other end of a phone call from your sister or best friend. So it upsets you to hear that I'm in pain or that I'm scared of dying. We've only just begun our virtual best friendship; you're not ready for it to end.

I wish we had met under different circumstances, perhaps a fashion or gossip blog. But unfortunately that's not where my life path took me. I still hope to prove those doctors wrong, but I can't go along pretending like nothing's happening. For starters the pain wouldn't let me! As hard as this may be for you, just imagine how hard it is for the thousands of cancer patients going through this disease, their family and friends. If you can feel this emotionally connected to essentially a complete stranger, imagine how their hearts are breaking.

One thing's for sure, whenever I do finally kick the bucket, I'll have way more friends, both virtual and real, going out than I did coming in. I receive daily prayers and support from thousands of you Fabulous Rockstars, and that gives me comfort that I never thought I would have. I am so thankful for all of you and your genuine concern. You take the time out of your day to read my biblical-sized blogs, and then you make loving comments. My family, friends and I are so thankful that you feel I'm worth that time and energy.

Lisa's virtual friends never fail to surprise me. They remained loyal throughout her illness and continue to stay loyal today. Not a day goes by without someone messaging, just to check in on Peter, me and our family. They continue to offer support in many ways. If it's not offering up a special prayer for us, it's to send some soothing oils or some beautiful words they believe will comfort us. It's no different to when Lisa was with us. Like the family, some struggled more than others to accept that cancer would eventually kill Lisa. They were very similar to our family when Lisa was originally diagnosed as terminal. We believed as did Lisa that a cure or a miracle would happen, and that Lisa would live a long happy life.

> She never believed she would die.

Lisa confirmed this a few days before she passed. She never believed she would die.

An Indescribable Love

12/12/2016

As you all know, I wasn't blessed with children. I've often questioned whether I have experienced the deepest love a person can experience in their lifetime. Yes, I'm a daughter, a sister, a granddaughter, an aunty and so on. I know I'm loved, and I love them. But is our love for each other as deep as a love for a partner or your own child?

I've been in love. I know what that feels like, and it compares to no other love, well, any love that I've had. There's something special about a loving relationship, a feeling that is pretty indescribable. But I can say it's a deep and unwavering commitment to another soul. When I've been in the depths of my deepest love with a partner, it's like I walk around with love blinders on. I would walk in front of a speeding train to save them. I've felt that, and it doesn't compare to a love you have for your parents or siblings. It's no more important; it's just a different type of love. When it hits you, you'll know because it's both exhilarating and scary. Scary? Yes, because you're in so deep you're frightened something might take that away from you. You're scared they don't feel the same, and that it won't last or it's not real.

As I thought about the different types of relationships in my life and the type of love we have for one another, I had a realisation. All this time I've worried about how much people love me, how much people will miss me and what impact I have had on their lives. I especially worry about Ava. You see everyone else has had time to love me, to make lasting memories with me, but Ava? Well, she's only three. So I worry that when I do kick the bucket, she might not be old enough to remember our relationship. Yes, we've made memories. Yes, we've developed a loving relationship. Even though she's going through the terrible threes now and she's more unpredictable than a USA election, we still have what I believe to be a very special bond.

This evening Ava told me she doesn't love me because I was mean to Nanna. But moments before she was following me everywhere and I turned around and said jokingly, "Ava, stop following me," to which she replied, "But Lisa I'm only following you because I love you". That kid is like having a shower with the dishwasher on at the same time. She goes from hot to cold and back again in seconds, but I love her.

So my lightbulb moment? I've always thought that no matter how special these relationships, I'm leaving no-one behind. More specifically, I'm not leaving a child behind – another one of those bonds that people say is like no other. In fact, many say there is no deeper a love than the love you have for your own child. But then I thought about the love I have for my Aunty Bernie.

So why my Aunty Bernie? Why did she stand out? I have one of those loves for my aunty that's unlike any other love I have for anybody else. I used to basically live at her house when I was a kid. My other aunties have so many nieces and nephews that it all gets a bit diluted, whereas my Aunty Bernie only had me and my brother. So it always felt special. Bernie is one of the kindest souls you'll ever meet. She is so devoted to myself and my family that she has dropped everything and flown out here to Australia a few times in recent years to support my family and get us through the hard times. There are times she's been sitting on a plane not knowing if I'll be dead or alive upon her arrival. Can you imagine that feeling? Bernie has gotten me through so many low moments over recent years. She is a beacon of light for all of us in our darkest hour, but especially for me.

We didn't always have this relationship. I'm sure there were a few times she probably would have killed me after catching me going through her Fine Young Cannibals or Boy George records when I was a kid. If it weren't for the high probability of jail time, I probably would have been wearing concrete shoes at the bottom of some lough in Ireland years ago. God, I was scared of her as a kid! She was certainly a fiery one in her early twenties. But as we both grew up we grew closer, even if we were thousands of miles apart. Our love and admiration for each other has grown and continues to grow with each day. Bernie has a husband and a son now. I'm so happy for her as she deserves to love someone in that indescribable way, and someone deserves to be loved by her in that indescribable way too.

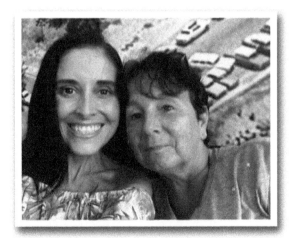

4 February 2017
Lisa and her Aunt Bernie.

If I can have that love and commitment for my aunty, an indescribable love, a never-ending love, then surely if I can manage to stick around long enough, Ava can have an indescribable love for me too. I know my love for her is already indescribable. I don't have to have a husband or a child to experience deep love or be loved deeply in return. I'm surrounded by indescribable love.

I'm surrounded by indescribable love.

To all my aunties, my love for each of you is indescribable.

To my uncles, my love for each of you is indescribable.

To all of my family and friends, my love for you is indescribable.

In the end, I'd say that's a pretty special thing, to know that you've loved indescribably and that you've been loved indescribably. Even if you think you haven't, when you sit back and think about it, you probably already have.

Stay Fabulous, Rockstars.

I wish Lisa could see the love that Ava has for her still, which continues to grow every day. Her memories of Lisa are vivid and each of them are special. As far as Ava is concerned, no-one will ever fill Aunty Lisa's shoes. She loves her unconditionally. There are many times she will climb onto Lisa's bed just to have a chat with Lisa's 'angel house' (her urn). She will tell her about special days that are planned and whispers a secret or two. Her conversations always end the same. "I love you Lisa and I want you to come back from heaven, so I can give you a big hug."

There are times when our chats about Lisa will lead to a few tears, especially now that Ava is beginning to understand the meaning of forever. I think she had this thought in her head that Lisa would eventually come home from heaven. Only yesterday Ava asked how Lisa got a sore tummy. I tried to describe it as simply as possible, but the how's and why's continued. I expect this will continue to be a question we'll revisit time and time again. One thing is for sure, though, Ava knows how much she was loved by Lisa. And the love that Ava has for Lisa is just as strong. Lisa will never be forgotten.

As for my sister Bernie, Lisa is so right. She was there throughout our nightmare journey. We just had to say the word and she was here. She held us all together when we felt we were falling apart, and she always had the right words at the right time. Lisa's love and admiration for her were endless. As a family at the other side of the world we were lucky. We had so much love and support from those near and far.

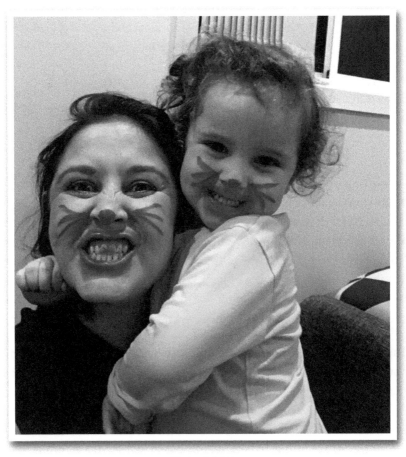

28 April 2016
Lisa and Ava at home having lipstick fun!

TERMINALLY *fabulous*

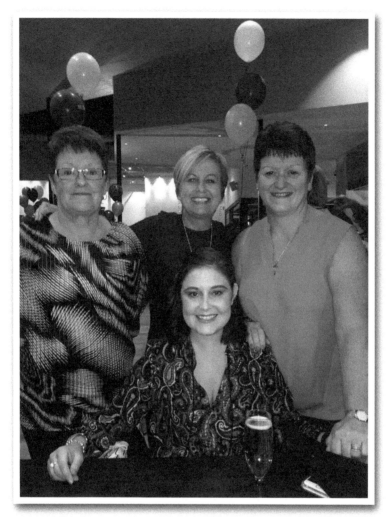

4 July 2016
Aunties Pauline Murray and Teresa McDermott with Lisa
and Geraldine at Orion Hotel, Springfield Central.

Gaunt and Bloated

18/12/2016

So here I am, and I've just looked at my reflection in the mirror. For months now I've been going on ad nauseam about my bloated, double-chinned, Bert Newton-Amanda-Vanstone's-love-child face. But tonight I am looking emaciated and gaunt with eyes sunken. I am looking more and more like a contestant on *Survivor* every day. It's horrible.

Around the time of the Cup, I was starting to feel more human, more like myself facially. I wasn't quite there, but I was starting to get my groove back. Here I am six weeks later, and I still look six months pregnant from tumours, tumour fluid, bloating and my good old friend constipation. My thighs remain bloated from medication, but the rest of my body is losing weight, and losing it quicker than a celebrity mum loses her post baby weight.

I know what you're thinking: *You can't win with this girl.* Well, all I want is to be somewhere in the middle, just plain old average. I don't want to be a bloated mess and I don't want to be a skinny wreck. I'm tired of wasting meals that my mum puts great effort into making. As soon as I take the first bite, I'm trying to push back the urge to regurgitate. I force myself through half a meal most times, but by the time I've gotten comfortable on the lounge after dinner, I've got mum or dad running for a sick bag. Or I'm hobbling to the toilet, trying to avoid a scene from the *Exorcist,* without the head turning and demonic possession. Is it really too much to ask to at least look a little normal on the outside when the insides look like a scene from a *Saw* movie? I'd just like a nice happy medium.

I remember the last time I had major issues like this. It was days before I was going under the knife for the fifth time. I remember I was on holiday up north with my ex. I had been admitted to Cairns emergency where they inserted a NG tube whilst I was awake, with no local. That would have been my third or fourth. The NG tube is inserted so you can receive liquid food rather than eating it. They put an 11-millimetre tube up your nostril and feed it down your oesophagus until it hits your stomach. (I've had one go into my lung by mistake before; that wasn't fun.) The problem is, when they're feeding this plastic tube down your nose, you have a bunch of food that hasn't been digested sitting in your stomach, so it makes you sick. At the same time as the nurses are telling you to swallow the tube, you're trying to get rid of the vomit. Definitely not pleasurable, but I've become really good at them over the years. I don't even gag anymore. I know, such an achievement.

When I came out of the mammoth eight- or nine-hour surgery, my colorectal surgeon, whom they called in mid-surgery as it was more detailed than they thought, told me I'd have had days if I was lucky. There were tumours throughout that were just about to cause major blockages. Without that surgery, I probably wouldn't have been alive the following week.

Here we are again, in the same pain, the same discomfort as that February back in 2014. But this time, I have no back-up plan, no contingency. So not only am I shit-scared I'm going to have a major blockage and die, I'm also scared I'm going to die gaunt and swollen. Just give me a break.

My poor niece Ava had to witness me once again collapse to the ground writhing in pain, trying to catch my breath to scream for someone to inject me with my pain med. I was upstairs, and Mum, Dad and Ava were outside in the backyard. Mum heard me after what felt like an eternity but would only have been a minute. Mum was yelling, with Ava likely watching on in horror, trying to locate where in the house I was. Mum found me and injected my meds. In the meantime, I could hear Ava sort of sobbing behind Mum, pretend sobbing I think. It's not right that a three-year-old should have to witness her aunty so feeble and weak. Shortly after Ava came over to me and asked if I was fine as I normally soothe her, telling her, "It's fine, Bubba" when I'm having a painful episode. But I didn't soothe her this time, so I think she needed reassurance.

I told her I was fine, and Ava promptly went to the backyard and told Mum in a stern authoritative voice, "Lisa is NOT fine, Nanna".

As I sit here and type and bitch and moan at 1am, I'm reminded of a beautiful message I received from a work colleague from way back. She mentioned that a person had come into her workplace and was going through cancer. My workmate mentioned me and the blog, and to her surprise the person said she reads my blog and it keeps her focused. Such a very small thing in such a very big world. It just shows you that you can touch a person's life without even knowing. You can give them a source of comfort and help in their healing, all without meeting. This made my heart sing, to know that this interaction had happened at the

> You can touch a person's life without even knowing.

opposite end of the country whilst I was probably brushing my teeth or watching *Housewives of Something* somewhere.

Such a small interaction in such a big world, and it has made my week. It still doesn't change the fact that I'm pissed off I can't keep a sip of water down. But it's something nice to think about when my head is in the loo.

To a random person with this horribly random disease, thank you. I can't promise things will get better or worse but know that you certainly made me smile. And 'workmate', you know who you are, thank you for being the messenger.

I hope you're all having a wonderful weekend, filled with tinsel and Christmas-inspired coffees and cocktails.

And of course, stay Fabulous, Rockstars.

It was becoming more and more evident that Lisa was steadily declining. Her good days were rare, and for the first time in a long time, even make-up couldn't hide the damage that cancer was doing to Lisa's body. It was heart-wrenching to watch.

Christmas was around the corner, and as a family we went through the normal pretence. We pasted on our Christmas smiles. My stomach was in constant knots, and Peter was beginning to discuss what lay ahead of us. He could no longer hide from the inevitable. I wanted to close my eyes at night and wake up after Christmas. I didn't feel like I could deal with any more emotions. You see, Christmas was Lisa's favourite time of the year. She was always so excited in the lead-up to Christmas. Even though she'd had the worst three years of her life, she still managed to have the best wrapped Christmas presents around the tree. No matter how ill she was, she would not let cancer ruin it for her.

I wish the same could be said for me. Three years prior, we were told to make the most of Christmas as it would be Lisa's last. This year I didn't need to be told, and it was unbearable. Lisa looked so weak. Every day was a difficult day. All I could do was pray that the end was near. When I woke from what little sleep we managed to get, I just wanted to see her at peace and out of pain.

Will This Be My Last Visit from Santa?

22/12/2016

Life, you are like a boyfriend to me. I fucking love you. I would literally push a baby out of my five-cent-piece-sized LOVE hole for you, and then the next minute I hate you and wouldn't even turn your burning fish fingers over in the frying pan for you. There are times I'd happily take pictures with you and post them on Facebook, being all braggy about how good you are to me. The next day I'm gonna be taking those loving Life pictures down because you're so horrible to me.

> Life, you are like a boyfriend to me. I fucking love you, and then the next minute I hate you.

This is seriously what life with terminal cancer is like, particularly towards the latter end of the disease. The good days become fewer and the bad days become more common.

The unpredictability of this disease can be somewhat confusing to people who've never been affected by this disease or another terminal illness. One of the most difficult things people find hard to grasp is that I can be out and about, with it all hanging out, on Saturday. Then I'd be bedridden, in crippling pain, regurgitating everything that passes my lips and nauseated beyond belief from Monday for four consecutive days. And then I'd be up and about with it all hanging out again and repeat.

This is just how this disease works, especially with my tumours being throughout my abdomen and pelvis. My bowels are constantly moving, meaning my tumours are constantly moving. This also means poo is a big issue, especially if I get backed up. I've had major issues with pooing all my life, even before my disease. Throw in scar tissue, throw in pain and sickness meds that constipate you, and this is why my pain goes from a four to a ten in moments. Right now, for example, I've got pain in my lower right back from my liver tumours, which only arose two hours ago. Prior to that I hadn't had this type of pain in months. This might help people maybe understand a little bit more as to why I go into hiding for days at a time, and my hideouts are becoming increasingly more common and longer.

Today I had a great day. I'd pooed over the last few days (YAY!!!! Roll out the toilet paper, flush that loo, and let's celebrate!) and I was drinking water without it regurgitating. Then this evening after dinner, incredible nausea came over me. I was sweaty and hot but unable to vomit. It's just a horrible feeling that comes over you without the actual vomiting to make you feel better. I've become a cry baby of late. I just get to a point of sickness that the tears start rolling. My dad's asking if he can help. No, he can't. How can you help nausea, watching on helplessly as your daughter breaks down? That was it: needle time!

I have a nausea injection called cyclazine, which literally burns my flesh. It causes a build-up of blood under the skin and large lumps all over my arse. It's got to the point that we're running out of space to inject. You can't do it too close to the crack as you can hit the sciatic nerve, which I can't imagine being fun.

The injection is so painful, when it hits certain spots I cannot help screaming in pain. Both Mum and Dad did an injection separately. As they injected, my butt was so hard the syringe burst off, the medicine spurted all over each of them and the needle remained hanging in my arse. All three of us dread that evening injection. I think both of them literally hide until I've found the other to give it to me. I was informed today that my arse is just one big abscess waiting to happen. It's no wonder the boys are knocking my door down ... sarcasm. So we're looking at other options for the cyclazine to be administered.

So things have not been the best the past few weeks. But I have to believe that I will have an 'up' soon' because we've had too many consecutive 'downs' of late. I'm not being alarmist and I'm not writing this for attention or sympathy. I'm writing my truth and my thoughts down for you to read, not to judge me or feel sorry for me. That ain't my bag.

My honest truth at the moment is that this will be my last Christmas. As hard as that is for you to read, as hard as that is for my family to read, just imagine how hard it is for me to write – someone that has never believed "You're not going to make it to blah blah blah". Even when they said I wouldn't make it to Christmas in 2014, as upset as I was, deep down I just believed I would make it and it wouldn't be my last. I'm the person that calls Life her boyfriend and isn't ready to break up yet. Sadly, it seems my boyfriend is going to get in there first and dump me. I just hope he isn't a cheap bastard and at least holds out to this Christmas and my birthday!

Where are we right now? Fuck knows. I'm more confused than a hermaphrodite bi-sexual with gender dysphoria. Unfortunately, when you're diagnosed with terminal cancer, you're not given an instruction manual. You might get a crappy two-page printout from some cancer clinic, but each disease is different. Everybody's demise is different. I just fucking hate that I know mine isn't too far away. Nobody deserves this, nobody. Not me, not anyone.

At a time of year that I'm usually bouncing off the walls, driving everybody crazy with Christmas music and movies, I'm starting and ending most days in tears. This isn't me; it's never been me. Throughout this whole shit fight I've never been a sooky lala, but lately I've become one.

There are so many fears that come with this disease, and those fears change each day. Every day a new fear arises. Like today, I thought to myself about how frigging difficult a person I am to live with. With this illness comes a highly compromised immune system, meaning if I see you wipe your nose, I'm immediately asking for blood tests proving that you don't have a cold. If you have the runs, you're out and so on. It's happened to me before: a simple cold for you can become an ICU visit for me, with my blood pressure not going above 70 and a fever of 41 degrees Celsius. A doctor enters the room and tells you that you're probably not going to be around much longer, all from a common bloody cold.

Whilst yes, getting a cold and dying is a fear, it's not the one I'm talking about My fear is that I am so much hard work, this disease is so much hard work, that when I'm gone and the funeral dust has settled, that my loved ones will sit back and think *As sad as all this shit is, it's nice to finally be able to sit and take a breath and relax, without listening out in the background for Lisa to yell out for something.*

> I'm scared they'll
> feel relief.

I'm scared they'll feel relief.

With all this crap I write, you all must think I want people to build shrines to me, get me cryogenically frozen, sit me in place of the TV and basically wear black every day mourning me until their time comes. But I don't want that. I would never want that. I simply want to be remembered for my good side – for the love I had for friends, family and life. Not for my shitty, bitchy side, which has been much more prevalent of late.

If I could have one Christmas wish, it would of course be the obvious: a cure for myself and for everyone suffering, and that no-one ever has to suffer again. Eradicate this bastard. Whilst many of you are wishing that your credit card bill had a couple less zeros on it, or that you could win the Lotto, here I am literally wishing for another Christmas after this one. Spare a thought for those that are doing it worse than you this Christmas. No matter how bad life is, there's always someone out there worse off than you and me.

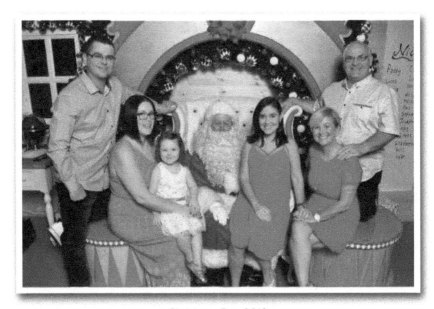

Christmas Day 2016
Annual Santa photo – Steven, Marianne, Ava, Santa, Lisa, Geraldine and Peter.
This was Lisa's last Christmas and she knew it. We all did and it was devastating. Still, we all put on a brave face.

Sooky lala signing off for now. I hope your week has been more kind to you.

Stay Fabulous, Rockstars.

Dying is Not Fun

07/01/2017

Crying has become more frequent, fear has become more ferocious and pain has become a part of daily life. Discomfort has become almost unbearable due to my bloated stomach suffocating my lungs and my bloated legs feeling like I'm walking on pain-sensored cushions. More food is coming back up than going down. My appearance could be best described as an eight-month pregnant skeleton with tree stumps for legs.

Doesn't that just wanna make you present right, boys?

So it would seem this bastard has got me. I have fought since September 2013, from the very moment I was told it was back and I would be lucky to make months. I fought, and I fought hard. Every time I was told you won't see tomorrow, you won't see Christmas, I defied the odds and a few clinicians had to eat their words.

I've tried my hardest to outrun this bastard, but not this time. It seems that damn shoelace I tripped over at the 10-kilometre line has allowed my killer to catch up. I can feel the air at my back from him swooshing his scythe at me, and I'm quite certain one day soon he'll get me. I simply don't have the confidence this time that things will get better.

They're not.

They're remaining the same, or in fact getting worse.

It's been a terribly steep decline in the last few weeks. I feel like I'm in one of those luge things from the Winter Olympics, just racing downhill with little to no control over what happens and how fast I go. My disease is taking me on this ride with nowhere to go other than down. I keep getting told to embrace God or your faith and that this whole process will become easier.

If I don't accept Him into my heart now, I'm told He may not accept me into His when it's my time to knock on the pearly white gates. Yet another image that's been imprinted in my mind since I was a child.

I cannot help my fear, nor can I control it. Nor should people be judgemental about how 'I' deal with 'my' inevitable death. We are all entitled to deal with this in our own way. There is no right or wrong. If you think Reiki is your path to spiritual healing, good on you. Or if you're an atheist, who am I to judge you for not believing when I am unsure myself of my own belief. I know what I want to believe, and I so greatly want this unwavering faith and confidence that it will come to fruition.

My symptoms are pretty much the same as they were on Sunday: big swollen legs from the cancer stealing my protein from me, causing fluid retention, a stomach full of cancer and this time bloated with a lot of ascites – a fluid that builds up due to the disease. There's so much fluid that when I inject my pain relief, it pierces little holes, allowing fluid to escape. It doesn't stop leaking; it just keeps going like piercing a water bed. I can't eat without regurgitating, and my cancer is eating all or any of my nutrients that I'm lucky to ingest.

I know I'm dying. I still haven't accepted it, and I'm still scared shitless. But I know I'm closer to death than I've ever been before. This death doesn't just affect me though. It affects all those around me, you Fabulous Rockstars and others that I come in contact with daily.

When I was in the hospital, I was surrounded by death. On one occasion I was informing my family that the young guy next door had died overnight and that a lot of the patients were dying. Next thing Ava speaks up. "Are you dying, Lisa?" I didn't know whether to just bite the bullet and I looked at her mum and dad to try to sense what they were feeling.

> I'll be a star and I'll make sure you'll never be scared.

But I just blurted out, "Yes, Bubba, Aunty Lisa is going to die. But remember when I do, I'll be up in the sky at night. I'll be a star and I'll make sure you'll never be scared". Ava listened intently and then she nervously giggled and replied, "You're silly, Lisa."

"Why?" I asked

She replied, "No Lisa you're not going to be in the sky because you're going to get better. I want you to get better, so you won't be a star". Out of the mouths of babes as they say.

I'm now at home struggling every night to organise my pillows and myself into a semi-comfy position in bed that lets me breathe, doesn't make me regurgitate as much, and allows me to elevate my legs for the swelling and so on and so on. Thank God I don't have a boyfriend. My pillows would seriously see more action than he would.

My bestie Rebecca and her housemate Chuck from Sydney dropped in and spent a couple of nights. Bec and I did our usual – talked for 10 hours and then realised it's bedtime. My friend Nicole popped in, also from Sydney, and I got to play with her baby girl and bitch about all the things we hate about humanity. That's what Nicole and I do. We have done it since she found out that I had been intimate with my first boyfriend, which she thought was hilarious at the time. Unfortunately, I ended up paying for our long talk, and I am physically and emotionally drained. I have now asked Mum to give me a week without visitors as I end up doing more than I should. I know I'm like the Queen. I request an audience when I want one.

It's amazing how the world listens sometimes. You ask and you shall receive. As I was tapping away at this blog, I received a phone call from my pall doctor. (She's amazing by the way.) She advised me that I was able to get my pelvic ascites drained in hospital on Monday, and to prevent having to be admitted again I can have a semi-permanent catheter inserted. This means that when the fluid returns, I can drain the fluid from home. We think there'll be about 7 to 8 litres drained over a couple of days in hospital. So I'm hoping this will ease my current discomfort.

Anyway, my friend Bec gave Mum and I a Worry Doll each. You tell her your worries, put it under your pillow and it takes your worries away. Mum being mum, she heard 'Wish' doll, so the following morning Miss Ava was in Mum's bedroom and saw the doll. Ava asked Mum what the doll was, and Mum replied, "It's a wish doll, Bubba. You tell it your wish and it will grant it". Ava picked the doll up and said, "I wish that my Nanna was happy, and that Lisa's belly gets better". That kid just rips my heart out.

So Fabulous Rockstars, at the beginning of this blog I was down and out, and by the end, although I'm still in the exact same discomfort, my hope has improved. Maybe we can all learn something from this. Dad, I promise I'm not ready for palliative sedation yet.

Stay Fabulous, Rockstars

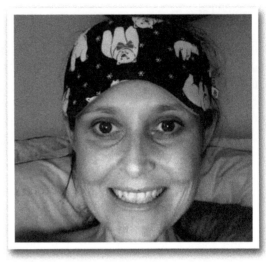

7 January 2017
Lisa

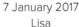

As much as Lisa was relieved about getting the drain fitted to her stomach, I had mixed feelings. A drain would mean another open wound and another opportunity for infection to kick in. It would also mean another process to learn, which we did not feel equipped for. I absolutely wanted Lisa to be more comfortable. She was literally trailing her poor body around, and other than her swollen stomach and legs, every other part of her body was skin and bone. Every footstep caused her pain. And then there was the pain on top of pain, which would cause her to drop to the floor until enough pain relief was given to give her the strength to get back up again. It was so cruel to watch. Our family were living on a knife's edge.

Through it all, Lisa kept fighting.

On Christmas morning Lisa got up, showered and put on her beautiful red-and-white Christmas dress along with her make-up. She looked absolutely amazing. The dress covered the heartbreak that hid behind every smile. Our gorgeous girl was dying yet she was determined that cancer was not going to ruin her favourite day of the year. However, by 11pm her pain and discomfort could no longer be camouflaged and by 12am we were back in emergency. These occurrences were becoming more regular, and with each visit Lisa's will to live became stronger but our ability to cope became weaker.

Thinking back, the week Lisa went in to get the drain fitted was one of the worst weeks I'd had throughout Lisa's cancer nightmare. Peter and I were taking turns sleeping in with Lisa and it was taking its toll. She was constantly coughing, regurgitating or crying out with pain, but nothing could keep her in bed to rest. Thinking back, why would it? She couldn't lie down, so how could she rest? Her body wouldn't let her.

I found myself suggesting that I sleep in Ava's room as it was the room next to Lisa's. This was not because I wanted to get some sleep but because I was struggling watching Lisa suffer 24/7. Subconsciously, I was pulling away and I couldn't help myself. As her mum I wanted to be there, needed to be there, but mentally I wanted to be as far away as possible. I feel great shame even writing this, but Lisa promised warts and all, and these are my warts.

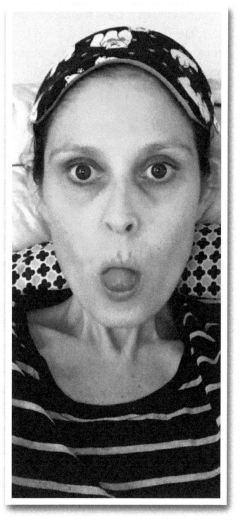

7 January 2017
Lisa

As much as Lisa understood me wanting to sleep in Ava's room, I could tell she was frightened. What if I didn't hear her? What if she choked on her vomit and couldn't breathe? Why didn't I just go in? No matter how hard

I tried, I couldn't. I was falling apart at the seams, frightened this would go on forever and frightened it wouldn't. It was then I decided to go see my doctor to get my antidepressant medication reviewed. It was evident that I wasn't coping.

On the morning we were going into get the drain fixed, Lisa was extremely agitated with me. We were unsure if she would be coming home that night or would have to stay at the hospital. When I entered her room, she had already started packing but was clearly upset at having to do it herself. I started to help, but she was getting more annoyed. I left the room and went to get her medication organised. When I went back to her room, Lisa became extremely aggressive. I suggested she sit down and tell me what to put into her case, but she was that frustrated and in pain by this stage she told me I was a f@*$ing useless carer and never to think about taking it up as a career. I honestly couldn't say exactly what else was said as I was struggling just to keep myself upright. I got Lisa's sickness injection ready (yes, the one that went into her bottom). With a lot of resistance Lisa finally agreed to let me give it to her.

By the time we were driving to the hospital, I was choking on the lump in my throat. I will never know how I drove the car that morning without getting us killed. Lisa tried to engage in conversation about what had been said and demanded that we speak about it before we get to the hospital. My only response was to tell Lisa that the one thing she couldn't control was when I was able to talk.

You can imagine how tense things were by the time we reached the palliative ward. It was so evident that one of the beautiful nurses stopped me to ask if I was okay. That's when the tears came and wouldn't stop. In my head I knew Lisa loved me and was taking her frustrations out on me. But in my heart, I was hurting. In a way I knew Lisa was right. I wasn't a carer. I was a mother who was watching her only daughter dying in one of the cruellest ways, and there was nothing I could do about it. By the time Lisa went to get the drain fitted, we were both in tears. Lisa was apologising time and time again, and I was crying so hard with a pain in my heart I thought would never go away.

For the first time in a long time, I didn't stay with Lisa in the hospital that night. This wasn't to make her hurt or pay for what she had said but to clear my head before my doctor's appointment the next morning. I just needed to get my thoughts together and to reenergise before Lisa came home the following day. Needless to say I didn't get a lot of sleep that night as I was riddled with guilt and a feeling of unease. But that was nothing new.

During my appointment with my doctor, she recognised our need for additional support. Discussions around getting a nurse to help us at home were instigated with palliative care. Palliative care also suggested that Lisa stay in the palliative care ward and go home for a few days a week. But Lisa wouldn't hear of this. She wanted to be at home, and as hard as it was I fully understood this. What I didn't know nor understand was where I was going to find the strength to keep going.

Thankfully, Peter could see my desperation and he took two weeks off work to give me a break. As crazy as it must sound to someone who has never dealt with this situation, I really don't know how I'd have coped otherwise.

A Little White Lie

18/01/2017

A short blog for a short update. ♡ 🤘

Last night I was faced with a dilemma. You see, I've been placed back in hospital, back to the ward that insists they're there to make you feel comfortable and to try to reduce symptoms and pain. They are not always there to prepare you for the scariest time in a person's life. I don't give a shit if you say this is not scary and is simply part of the process of life. We all live knowing eventually we will die. Blah blah. Well, yeah, we all live knowing at some point we're probably going to need root canal therapy, but I've never seen anyone skip into a dental surgery.

Too sick to cry, too weak to move, constantly vomiting bile, too weak to get myself out of bed, down the stairs. Too weak to get in the car, too many tumours to pee and the list goes on. My pall nurse made me come in and she inserted the urinary catheter, always a pleasant experience.

Yesterday I looked, but more importantly felt, that I was at death's door. I've been at so-called 'deaths door' so many times that they know it's me by my knock. But I've never actually felt that my body was giving in. I never believed it was 'my time'. Last night came and it was time for people to say goodbye. With more than generous bear hugs from each of my family members came that so-called dilemma, "I'll see you tomorrow".

My reply: "Yep, I'll see you tomorrow."

> Tomorrow is
> not a promise
> - it's a gift.

My actual thought: "Will I really see you tomorrow?" ... something we say every day without a second thought, because hey, tomorrow is taken for granted. I hate to be the bearer of bad news, but sadly tomorrow is not a promise – it's a gift. And that's only if you're lucky enough to receive it.

It's a frigging horrible feeling to say goodbye to someone you love and not know if you'll ever see them again. I only wish for you, Fabulous Rockstars, that you never have to be placed in a situation like this. It's truly one of the most heart-breaking places to be, and nobody deserves that. Make sure your hugs are genuine and so too is your love.

Stay Fabulous, Rockstars. ♡ ✌

If only I'd known how Lisa felt about being left alone that night. That's the problem. As much as I know there was absolutely nothing I could do to change the fact I was truly struggling at this stage, I'm now left with the 'what ifs'. How could I have left her at such a critical time in her illness? Please try not to judge me for my actions. I was doing my best. Only people that have walked a day in my shoes will truly know what I was going through at this stage.

Just an Update

24/01/2017

To all my loved ones, friends, Fabulous Rockstars, 'my ride or die' so to speak, I'm still going. I'm just not going at the speed of a fully-functioning Fabulous Rockstar. More Mick Jagger than Adam Levine, let's say.

I have been discharged from Palazzo Palliative, as you probably know. It has gotten to the point that my team believe more regular interludes in hospital would be beneficial, so we shall see how that pans out.

I am at the lowest I've ever been in my disease. I've been told I'm dying before, but now it feels like I'm dying. WTF. How would I know what dying feels like? I suppose I'm just guessing, but I'd say this is a pretty good guess of what it feels like.

Whilst in hospital I had a urinary catheter inserted, as I've said. I had to rush to the toilet to do number two's, so I grabbed all my bits and pieces, catheter, pain driver ... I was connected to the IV, so I was very weighed down. I jumped up and the next thing I felt like I'd been coat hangered. My catheter tube got caught around the end of the bed and I slammed face down onto the floor. I could hear Mum had run into the bathroom and was shouting. The emergency alarm was hit by my nurse and everyone ran from all angles. After assessing the situation they picked me up. The catheter had dislodged, and let's just say I was in a bit of pain. My ever-loving nurse removed the catheter for me and disaster was averted. But that makes it four times I've now popped a catheter balloon by pulling it out. Now that's skill.

Unbelievably, my bladder started working again. I must have nine bladders! Everyone expected I probably would be spending my remaining time in palliative and not getting back out. But I am now sitting in a holiday

> That first breath in the morning is fucking amazing.

259

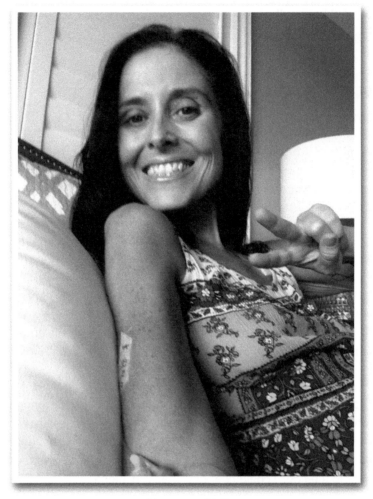

24 January 2017
Lisa relaxing by the sea at Broadbeach, Gold Coast, after another hospital visit.
We knew that Lisa's life was coming to an end. She was fading away in front of us.

house that my aunty and granny have organised. I went to bed to the sound of waves crashing on the shore last night. As I prayed to God to give me the strength I needed to wake in the morning, I woke to the same crashing waves. Life is beautiful and that first breath in the morning is fucking amazing.

I am probably under 30 kilos now, and my appetite and nausea does not allow for eating. Two mouthfuls and I'm done. I have been told to stop focusing on eating as loss of appetite is part of this process: you get tired, you lose appetite and then you pass. But seriously, who the fuck could just accept that? Stop eating, let yourself die. How about you stop showering, stop breathing?

I get it. What can you say to a person who is literally wasting away and dying before your eyes? See you on the flip side just doesn't seem to cut it.

Thanks for the love, Fabulous Rockstars. Please don't be concerned with my blog post intervals. I promise I'll keep you up to date, just not every day. Can I also ask that you spare a thought/prayer/vibe for my parents, loved ones and family? They're going through this journey just as I am.

Stay Fabulous, Rockstars. ♡ 🤘

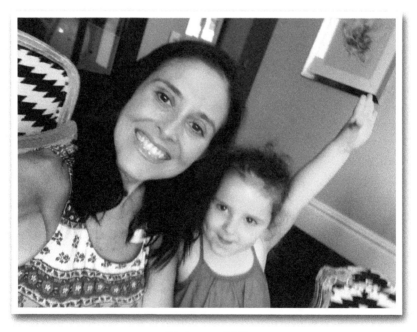

24 January 2017
Lisa and Ava at Broadbeach, Gold Coast. Selfie time!

This is a cruel disease. It strips you down to your bare bones, taking everything you have ever taken for granted with it. By this stage there was no sleeping, no eating, no energy. Lisa's organs were slowly shutting down and even breathing became a challenge. My head and heart continued to fight with each other, to let her go or make her comfortable enough to keep going. I couldn't do either of those things, but God could. And I questioned why He wasn't stepping in. Our discussions as a family had changed. We didn't talk about Lisa in the future any longer. We talked about how long we thought she could go on. I was no longer alone in these thoughts. Peter, Steven and Marianne knew it was just a matter of time.

World Cancer Day

13/02/2017

For the world, it's World Cancer Day. For me and many others, it's World Cancer Day 365 days a Year. A little blog on my current state and thoughts on today.

World Cancer Day, Lisa's every day, millions of other people's day. A day that some people may sit and reflect on the travesty that is this horrendous disease. Others may think about how lucky they or their family are for escaping or beating the disease. And then there are those that have no idea that it's even World Cancer Day.

I'm so disappointed. I was asked by the two fabulous queens – Queen Originalé herself Constance Hall and her best queen since kindergarten, Annaliese Dent – to go on their show *The Queen Sesh* to have a chat about the bastard that is cancer. I was very excited to do it, especially to get the rare cancer word out and, well, if I'm really honest, it was a good excuse to have a good bitch sesh with two of my faves.

Anyway, with this beast being the rollercoaster disease it is, I've been choking on vomit in the middle of the night. This is burning my oesophagus, causing pain, a husky voice, making my voice break and leaving me breathless. Needless to say I'm not up for doing my little segment, which pisses me off as I don't like to back out of anything. I'm sure I could do it, but if it's not great, I don't want to do it! The only thing I can take solace in is that there is now no risk of me stealing their show from them, which I'd hate to do. They were my two biggest backers in the beginning of my blog, and they didn't even know me. They just read the blog and had faith.

Love you girls more than the chicest pair of shoes ever featured in a *Sex and the City* episode. But remember, if you're going to buy me some, go half a size up. I honestly think red bottoms would cheer me up, no pressure ... Well, some. 😜👡👠👞👑

So, World Cancer Day is my EVERY day. It's not a day for a ribbon. It's not a day for remembering. Sadly it's my existence. Not being able to go on the radio show is one of those little annoying things that cancer gives. These little gifts individually may be annoying, but they build up. The unpredictability of this whole disease for me is something I don't think I'll ever get used to. So for those of you out there dealing with this disease, be prepared for losing control.

You lose control of your body, your strength, your appearance, your emotions and your mental ability. You can lose your vision and other vital organs or senses, your hair, weight, muscle density, bone density and so much more. It's at the point where I can't stand from a sitting position at a particular level without physical help. And I can only make five steps before my legs fall from under me on the stairs.

Losing predictability is one of the worst things. We predict we will wake up tomorrow. We predict we'll see our friends, family and loved ones again. But imagine if you were given a death sentence without a date, so that every day you know you could die. You know every day could be your last. You'd probably spend a lot of your time thinking, W*hen, where, how? Will I just have a massive bleed and die? Will my bladder stop and that's it? Stop eating, start sleeping constantly?*

Maybe it will be like now. My lungs have started aspiration. I got the results from my chest X-ray, which confirmed aspirated pneumonia. Now that's the type of shit that takes a weak one like me out. My docs are again not giving dates as I have always defied them, but "You could be around in four weeks or two" have been bandied around from a few different specialists, nurses and docs. When someone says you could be here in four weeks like it's God's greatest gift to man, it doesn't fill you with much confidence.

I get it. I've already squeezed three years out of a couple of days, but to me it's like if you buy a loaf of bread with a use-by date of six days from now and it remains fresh for nine days. Woopty fucking doo! Break out the party poppers and streamers, let's celebrate!!!! I know I'm being cynical and childish and selfish and any other word you can think of that means bratty. But four weeks is a fleeting holiday on the Queensland coast, not much of a remaining life.

I love that we as a 'world' reach out and show our support for cancer, in many different ways. There are so many different cancers, and that's why it makes it so difficult to cure. People often think one cure fits all, but that's like saying one pair of Christian Louboutin fits all. Well, as much as we try to squeeze our normal size 36 into one, you really need half a size up. Any girl worth her weight in shoes knows red bottoms usually run a bit small. Just like my favourite shoe, every cancer has a different genetic makeup or hormonal makeup. No one cancer is exactly the same, and that's why the 'elusive' cure has not been found yet.

> Cancer is like a dirty, stinky, unwashed c**t on a 40-degree day.

I was asked via FB messenger to describe cancer. Just a caution, this does involve language albeit with asterisks, but BAD language: Cancer is like a dirty, stinky, unwashed c**t on a 40-degree day.

They say everything happens for a reason and God only gives 'His' greatest battles to those who have the strength to fight them. But I'd really like to know what the prerequisites are for this selection process as I can't for the life of me, or in my case impending early death, figure out why I'd be selected as any stronger than some CrossFit fanatic that dreams of protein shakes and shits green daily because she lives on wheat grass and edamame. Wouldn't they be stronger?

I've asked this question before and the response from people is pretty much the same 9/10 times. Just because someone has a strong body doesn't mean they have a strong mind or the emotional gumption to persist with this unimaginable disease.

Please, cancer needs you. People like me need you, and the last thing we want to ask for is charity. But sometimes you gotta put your fedora where your mouth goes and shake it for a good cause.

I know a lovely Rockstar has started a GoFundMe for my family and I to raise money for a nurse at home on occasion and a stair seat lift as I'm carried upstairs now that I can't make it myself. But this isn't about me and my small picture. This is about the big picture of cancer on the world scale. So here's a few worthy charities for you to consider giving to today.

www.dreams2live4.com.au
www.rarecancers.org.au
www.cancer.org.au

Please do not feel obligated to donate. I just wanted to throw them in.

It seems very foreign to be saying "HAPPY WORLD CANCER DAY!" so I won't. I'll simply say "HERE'S TO LEARNING MORE ABOUT CANCER DAY AND RAISING FUNDS TO TRY AND FIX IT!!!!!"

Love you all more than gluten.

Stay Fabulous, Rockstars. ♡🤘👧

I remember seeing posts for World Cancer Day and collections taking place at our local shopping centre and after donating a few dollars, never giving it a second thought. It's not until cancer comes knocking on your door that you fully understand the impact and need for these amazing awareness days to continue.

Each minute of every single day was now a struggle. Lisa was so exhausted and yet so aware that it's just a matter of time. I was amazed she was able to write this blog.

Draining the stomach had now become an issue. As Lisa's stomach filled with fluid, her pain increased as the tumours were being moved around. The same thing happened when we drained the fluid. Her pain and discomfort increased and therefore the benefit was questionable. You're damned if you do and damned if you don't. My fear of cleaning the wound had also grown due to the ever-increasing risk of infection, which was becoming a major concern. At that time there was an extremely large green sore on Lisa's bottom caused by the burning of the sickness injections (cyclasine). So not only could Lisa not lie down because of the risk of choking and the pain caused by adding pressure to the tumours, but now sitting was also causing extreme pain.

Our doctor was great. She was coming and cleaning the wound and dressing it. But she recommended that we handle it with caution as we were unsure of how deep the infection went. So bursting the abscess could lead to bigger issues and the potential risk of spreading the infection. The underlying message was clear: Clean it, cover it up and don't mess with it. Keep it intact for as long as possible as Lisa doesn't have too long left and she has enough to deal with.

How do you comfort your daughter that things will be alright when you know it's far from alright? I picked my moments carefully to open up discussions with Lisa to prepare her for what lay ahead as no-one else could do it.

Taking When You Like to Give

13/02/2017

Just an update and a 'thank you', Fabulous Rockstars. ♡🤘

Thank you for the Love.

Taking money when you're not a taker, boy, is it hard. I've had terminal cancer for three years and five months. Over this time, I've been told I'm dying more times than people ask Sofia Vergara to repeat what she just said. Soooo when people have suggested fundraisers or money-raising efforts for me, I've always said thanks but no thanks.

As you all know, a few weeks ago I was once again admitted to palliative care in hospital. Deals were made for me to get out of hospital for a few days to visit the coast with my family from overseas. After a few days my body started to regain some strength. I was able to digest food (well, sort of) and take a crap. (Can I get a woot woot?) Other normal human body behaviours started to improve, so I was allowed to return home after the coast trip rather than to palliative care in hospital. Thankfully, since that last palliative visit, I have not had to return to the ward.

At that stage I was unable to even stand in the shower unassisted. I would walk up the stairs and my legs would collapse from under me at the top. Falling down became the norm. I was choking on my own vomit through the night. I do still regurgitate. I couldn't pee, and once again I was catheterised. I could barely eat or even stand the sight or smell of food. I lost a heap of weight. I still can't lie flat in bed and have to sit up to sleep. I couldn't reach to wipe my own arse. I had an incision made in my stomach in which a tube is inserted. Any tumour fluid or ascites that build up in the abdomen are then drained via the hole, hopefully alleviating the pressure and reducing nerve pain and some of the bloating. I read that people with tumour ascites usually have one week to a month to live. Hence, the reasons my medical team were a bit quiet on it. Who wants to tell a patient that type of news?

My mum, God love her, just doesn't have the upper body strength to assist me up the stairs or manoeuvre me in the shower or bath. Not that the bath thing matters as I can't have my stomach drain immersed in bodies of water. I'm also looking at a stair lift as my dad has bad arthritis. So even though he looooooves helping me up the stairs, there comes a point where you have to be honest with yourself and you need to accept help, just as I have had to accept you wonderful, giving Rockstars.

Things looking so bleak, I had to start to reconsider my death situation again. You see, originally, I had decided to just die in palliative care in hospital as I was still in my previous unhealthy relationship and it took that decision out of my hands. Now that I'm single, my true desire to die at home with my family can be achieved without fear or judgement. The only problem is that when it gets to that time, I would need a nurse here 24 hours a day. As you can imagine, that's definitely not what you'd call cheap. Whilst in hospital, it was discussed and suggested with palliative care that we should perhaps obtain the services of a stay-at-home nurse, especially to help Mum and

Dad with their at-home care. The poor bastards could enter *Married at First Sight;* that's how little they see each other now.

I wanted to do this update/blog as I want 100 per cent transparency. People hear 'stay-at-home nurse' and they automatically think of the patient and that things must be going downhill. But nurses aren't just for us. Yes, when discussing the hiring of a nurse a few weeks ago it was mostly for overnight stays as I choke at least three or four times a night. My vomit goes into my lungs, and if I'm not woken I'll die. My mum and dad have actually been sleeping with me every night. Yep, a 35-year-old woman and her parents in their early fifties are sharing the bed. The nurse is also there to ease the pressure on the carers and maybe give the carer a chance to get out for a haircut or a manicure. Maybe have a bath or, hell, maybe read a magazine from front to back.

Doctors and nurses are now cautiously saying that my situation is better than it was, meaning that I don't look like death warmed up anymore. But my disease is still everywhere and growing; that hasn't changed. The thing is my body seems to just keep fighting back. You start counting me out, my body becomes determined to prove you wrong. So even though I am currently suffering from the worst aspiration pneumonia I've ever had, all my stats say different. My oxygen levels are good, my lungs don't sound as wheezy etcetera etcetera. I'm defying odds and doing well again. But I can certainly say with all confidence that my body, although on the improve, is in its worst place, weakness wise, that it's ever been.

My pall team don't feel today that I need a nurse 24 hours like I did two weeks ago. But that's not to say I won't need one in three days' time for 24 hours. This disease is just so unpredictable. I am still trying to obtain a nurse for nights and a few days. The hardest part is someone to fill the position. When you're terminal, consistency is important. You don't want to have to go through your 6000 meds, allergies, back story and blah blah blah every goddamn nurse visit. The nurses can then administer my injections and IVs, change my wound dressings, drain my stomach and, most importantly, stay overnight to wake me and nebulise me when I'm choking. This means Mum and/or Dad can get more than an hour's sleep.

I want to say thank you to each and every one of you that has taken the time to donate your hard-earned money to a total stranger. I understand I have been very MIA of late, but my sickness is just consuming my thoughts at the moment. Although I think of you all numerous times a day, I just don't have the energy to read and reply.

I write my story for you, not for me or for financial gain. I write it so that you have someone you can relate to and to finally hear the reality that is cancer, not the cotton candy version.

I write my story for you, not for me or for financial gain.

To those of you who have written messages of support and those that donate five dollars and apologise, stop right now. Your words are enough. The fact that a single, unemployed mother is willing to give me the last of her very minimal pension, well, that just blows my mind. Those amazing people who have donated what some people would earn in a month's wage, thank you. Some people who I don't know that donate just read my blog. Others that I went to school with donate — both people who'd just say hi in the corridor and people who were the opposite of friendly too. It seems the people you would never expect would donate or send messages of love and admiration are the ones who are reaching out.

Either way, we will not have to cringe at the thought of opening bills for electricity that runs 24 hours a day because of my hot flushes, or pharmacy bills that arrive EVERY DAY because not everything is covered by PBS (Pharmaceutical Benefits Scheme). You have no idea how much this money will help. Cancer is a bloody expensive disease, especially if you keep punching it in the balls and defying the odds.

Thank you, thank you, thank you!

Margaret Hurd, thank you for ignoring my 'thanks but no thanks' to your offer to start the GoFundMe. Mum, thanks for managing messages and comments. I just don't have the energy at the moment to read and respond like I did a month ago. But each and every one of your comments still touch my heart, and my mum or dad read them for me, just as I've dictated this. Mum just luuurves writing about my vagina.

I may not have my health, I may not have my looks, and I may not have that quick wit that I used to pride myself on. But I do have you, each and every one of you Fabulous Rockstars. Now I'd say that's a pretty decent swap. Well, actually, I'd still prefer a cure for cancer. But for now, you guys will have to do!

Stay Fabulous, Rockstars. ♡

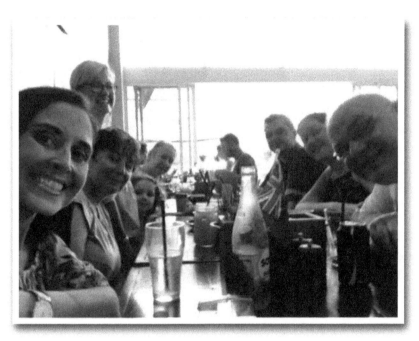

4 February 2017
A few nights with family at the Gold Coast, QLD. Lisa was
dying and she wanted to visit the beach one last time.

Up to this point, I'd been taking dictation intermittently but regularly for Lisa to post on the *Terminally Fabulous* blog. If her pain levels were too high, she was incoherent or couldn't focus, and then I was the typist. From this point on, though, she spoke and I typed. It was just too hard for her otherwise.

During this time, I was asked on numerous occasions how we felt about Lisa passing at home. I wasn't concerned about where Lisa passed. I was only concerned about whether we could control her pain levels. As much as Lisa wanted to be at home, the fear of her continuing to live in pain was unbearable. Although we had always resisted the offer of a GoFundMe page, the thought of having medical support at home and being able to go back to being Mummy rather than Carer meant more to me than our normally staunch pride.

One thing was for sure: my fear was at an all-time high. The only time I felt any kind of comfort was when Lisa was in hospital. Even though I was there with her 24/7, her medical needs were being met by the nurses, and decisions were being made by those qualified to do so. This was a massive relief to both Peter and me.

Timelines – Schmimelines

17/02/2017

A dear cancer blogger, someone whom I would like to say paved the way for the rest of us, was recently given the six-month timeline. *Dear Melanoma*, or Emma Betts, is first and foremost not a blogger. Emma is not her terminal melanoma diagnosis. She is a top chick with a huge heart. She gives even though life has taken so much from her. She gives care packages to people who are going through their own troubles. She messages me when she is in Emergency with her own problems to see how I'm doing. Emma is more than her cancer, more than her blog. If you're lucky enough to meet one person you admire, you'd be bloody lucky if it were her.

So six months. I remember initially I was told weeks or months, but I kept beating little milestones I would set for myself. With each treatment or surgery that would extend my life by mere months or even weeks, I would tick off invisible dates in my invisible calendar in my mind. I had myself dead in the first few days. I'm sorry to be so blunt, but that was the first thought I had because, in my initial diagnosis, everyone told me that if it came back I was incurable.

Just a bit of advice to any oncologists out there, new or long-term practising: DO NOT, I repeat, DO NOT advise a patient that has not even started treatment with you that, if this lifesaving toxic sludge they call chemo does not work and the cancer returns, they are incurable. That shit sticks in a patient's head like fake tan to a white pleather chair. Just keep your mouth shut unless you're asked a question. Don't answer, or of course feel free to offer considerate advice not stupid bullshit! This idiotic timeline hung around my neck like an invisible noose from the first ultrasound I had confirming my cancer's aggressive return. I was planning my funeral in the car trip home and crying that I'd never get to see my niece go to school or the next season of *Homeland*.

If you're in the your-cancer's-returned boat, remember to look around, visit different specialists and ask questions. Do all the things you probably didn't do the first time you were diagnosed because you just do what you're told the first time.

rarecancers.org.au have released an app called CAN.recall. It's a great tool for people having meetings with oncologists and surgeons. It gives you the best questions to ask, and it also records the session (at the specialist's consent, of course).

My point to this blog, which probably sounds familiar to many of my previous ones, is that timelines are time wasters. All they do is put invisible finishing lines at your feet. And even if they don't exist, you will keep tripping over them. So first things first. If you can, turn those death alarms off, put them on permanent snooze and live for tomorrow rather than waiting to die tomorrow.

All easier said than done, of course. People always ask me, "How do you stay so positive when you know effectively you're dying?" My answer is that I don't stay positive. The only thing that has kept me going mentally is the fact that I still don't believe it's happening. Somehow, I'm going to wake up tomorrow and it's all going to be gone. I've only just now had to start to realise that this shit is real. This breathlessness, this weight loss, this tumour fluid build-up in my stomach, this never-ending tiredness, loss of appetite and all of the other symptoms that are recognised as end-of-life symptoms are exactly that: I'm dying, sooner rather than later.

TERMINALLY *fabulous*

Six months shmix months, timelines shmimelines, doctors schmoctors, nurses schmurses. I've gone through more deadlines/timelines than Napoleon Perdis has gone through bronzer. We are all equal when it comes to living and dying.

I am still scared. I am still here, and for now, the four weeks mentioned last week are down to one week. More invisible timelines for me to ignore.

More invisible timelines for me to ignore.

Stay Fabulous, Rockstars. Let's not count down the deadlines together; let's ignore them together! ♡ 🤘

Emma, much love to you and yours. ♡♡♡

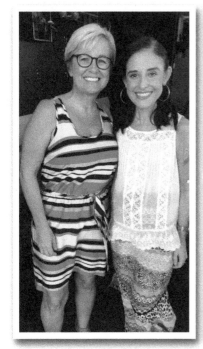
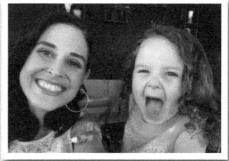
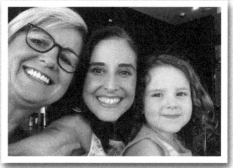

21 February 2017
Lisa spending cherished time with Geraldine and Ava at Lotus Cafe, Springfield Central, in her last ever outing.

Sadly, Lisa's friend Emma Simic (*Dear Melanoma*) passed away on Saturday 8th April 2017, four weeks after Lisa. She was 25 years old. Emma did so much work to raise awareness of melanoma whilst also raising funds for cancer research. Her parents Tamra and Leon carry on her work today. I know the two girls will be the best of friends up above – two beautiful angels taken way before their time.

As anyone that has lived through this hell will tell you, timelines are a real guessing game. As a parent, you just want answers. Somehow you think you can prepare better for what lies ahead, but the truth is ignorance is bliss. When I look back at what can only be described as an emotional rollercoaster, there is no way we could have kept going if we had placed any value on the timelines we were given. We'd have given up all hope three years ago.

The pressure put upon the medical profession to give families an idea of 'when' is so unfair. I know because I did it. They are not God. They see how you are hurting. They know the pain you are going through, and the last thing you need to hear is a best effort guess. Because that is all it is: best effort.

"What will be will be."

~Author unknown

Lisa's Final Blog

28/02/2017

Terminally Fabulous, you've made my life unique. I started this blog under a little duress, not to say that anyone can make me do anything I do not want to do. Gone are the days where I would choose clothes based on someone else's idea of what I should wear, even though it used to matter so much to me.

> *Terminally Fabulous, you've made my life unique.*

When I write that I was 'forced' into writing the

blog, it is more that I was convinced. I had a whole jinx thing going on in my head that if I start a blog, it might hurry my process along. I know it's a weird thought to have. I suppose I was concerned that bringing attention to my illness would bring other people with cancer or terminal illness to MY attention, and did I really want to get to know people that had the same fate as me? To make friends with people that were inevitably going to die and remind me that I was dying too?

You start a blog and people sometimes think you're some sort of authority on the topic. Believe me, just because Gwyneth Paltrow posts a paleo raw chocolate cake on her blog does not mean that she sources the ingredients and refines the technique and recipe. The thought that someone may write to me asking for advice about really personal and medical matters scares the shit out of me. I always tell people that I'm not an expert. I don't have a psychology or medical degree, so I never would give advice that could get you, or me, in trouble. Any thoughts I do give are my own, and I give them with love. Hopefully, they leave you feeling more heard and less confused and ignored.

I started writing this blog today because the fear I had about starting the *Terminally Fabulous* blog last February, and it making me accept my reality and face the pure scariness of it all, has come to fruition. I've made friends with strangers. We've built a community that supports one another, and in doing this I've let my walls down, in turn allowing this disease in and reminding me who's boss. As much as I want to stomp around acting like this cancer is my bitch, it's not. I am its bitch, and as the disease progresses, the tighter the restraints get.

I spend most of my days at home waiting for appointments that are basically the same meetings on replay. I sleep sitting up. I haven't lain down in at least four months. Bedsores are becoming a common fixture now. Sitting on my tailbone is like sitting on blades of glass. When my disease lets me, I go out. I eat when my disease lets me digest food. The disease dictates my days.

I'm writing today from a place of sadness. The fear of losing those I've connected with has started to become a reality, no longer a fear. People who've had terminal cancer the same or a similar length of time to myself are dying around me. We've been each other's supporters and listened to each other's fears, and now we're starting to drop like flies. I know we're not supposed to say, "This isn't meant to happen to us," and we're not meant to say things like "Bad things should happen to bad people". The truth is we don't believe that. We wouldn't wish this on our worst enemies. But sometimes we get so sick, so scared and so sad that we say things we don't mean. Having each other to say these things to in a safe environment, without feeling judged or wrong, is a large part of why we're there for each other.

Through this blog, I've known a few people now that have passed away. At the end of the day I suppose I can't write about all the fairy-floss-unicorn moments and ignore the more lifetime-movie-part moments that happen. THIS is my reality. Nothing can or will change that now. I am dying, just like them. No amount of pretending that I'm not will change that. I hate this disease. I hate that it's killing my friends and strangers, and I've had enough of thinking about it today.

Stay Fabulous, Rockstars ♥🤘

Unbeknown to Lisa, this was the last blog she would write. As the end drew near Lisa had us record her giving her beautiful *Terminally Fabulous* followers her final update. Every inch of her body ached, and her bodily functions were slowly and painfully shutting down. Instead of her beautiful 35-year-old immaculately made-up face, her face was sunken and etched with pain. Still, she found the strength to add humour and show love, gratitude and relentless dignity to those that had seen her through her darkest days – the amazing Terminally Fabulous Rockstars, all 67,000 of them.

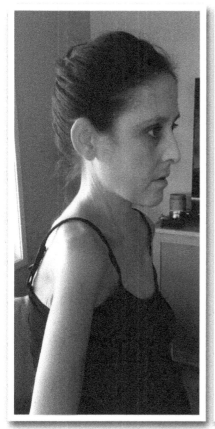

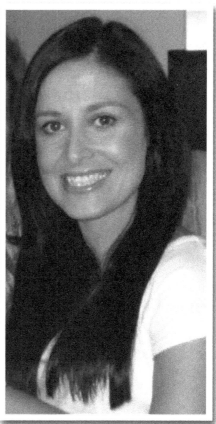

26 February 2017
Two weeks prior to Lisa's passing.

2011
Lisa pre-cancer.

When Losing Your Only Daughter Is the Best Option

"Your illness does not define you;
your courage and strength does."

~ Author unknown

2 March 2017

Waking to a loud bang, I jumped out of bed after a few hours' sleep. At only 35 years old Lisa was coming to the end of her cancer journey. Her main issues now were breathing difficulties and constant food regurgitation that caused her to choke throughout the night. If it wasn't food coming out her nose and mouth in her sleep, it was deep brown grainy blood. Sleeping propped up for the last six months had not helped, but it was all we could think of to try and minimise the risk of Lisa choking to death in her sleep.

By this stage, Peter and I were taking it in turns to sleep in Lisa's room. As her full-time carer some nights I just needed to be on my own to clear my head and re-energise for the next day. Watching her suffer was beyond unbearable. Knowing I could do nothing about it broke my heart.

Why did this evil disease have to be so cruel? Why couldn't it just allow our gorgeous girl a few hours' sleep? Why did her suffering need to be so relentless?

When I reached Lisa, she was lying on her bathroom floor with brown grainy fluid running from her nose. Her glazed eyes were open. Clearly, she had nothing left to give. Cancer had taken over every healthy cell in her body and was now trying to take her dignity. I hated this bastard disease.

Somehow, I managed to get her into the recovery position, although there wasn't much of her left. The cancerous fluid that consumed her body weighed her down and seeped through every pore. Getting hold of her without hurting her was impossible. Her temperature was high, and I knew I had to get her to the hospital even though this would go against her wishes. Her comfort was my priority. I wasn't just her carer; I was her mother.

I just knew this would be the last time Lisa would be carried out of our home by paramedics. If I'm being honest, I felt some relief. She had nothing left to give, and neither did we. Yet I also felt enormous guilt that I had let her down with her final wishes to pass at home. Either way, my first instinct as a mother was to get her out of pain and get comfortable, and this was no longer possible at home. All the love and best intentions in the world would never have compensated for the medical interventions needed.

By the time Lisa became coherent and comfortable in the hospital, our family had arrived at the hospital. Lisa being Lisa could tell what we were all thinking, but her determination shone through as always. She tried to reassure us that she'd be back on her feet in a day or two.

Despite deteriorating fast, over the next few days she continued to ask her palliative doctor when she would be going home. But by day three, I think she knew she would spend her final days in the ward she'd come to know so well. We were advised to tell family it was time to say our farewells. I don't know how we kept putting one foot in front of the other to get through this, let alone ring our nearest and dearest to share this devastating news.

For several days, there was a constant flow of people in and out of Lisa's room. There was laughter, tears and at times disbelief. Lisa had bounced back so many times before. Maybe she would do the same again. Our family GP had this very thought during her visit as Lisa was her witty, bossy and at times vibrant self. By the time she left, the doctor was quite confident she would be back doing her home visits to Lisa again very soon.

We were living at the hospital by this stage, frightened to go home just in case. Thankfully, our friends and family wouldn't leave us; they wanted to be close to us and Lisa. It was the only way we could get through.

Although Lisa was heavily medicated and fading in and out of sleep, she would rally and stay awake long enough to show us all that she hadn't lost her wit and sense of humour. Even in our darkest moments she had us laughing. She told us all that she loved us and hugged our three-year-old granddaughter Ava tight, not wanting to let her go.

Somehow, someway, Lisa was still with us one week later. She wasn't eating, and other than the odd sip of water she was barely conscious. Her organs were slowly shutting down. The only thing that awakened her at this stage was pain and discomfort. She'd often ask us to help her lie further up on the bed, but every touch was excruciating. When we did manage to get her propped up, she had no energy left to hold herself up and asked to be put back down again.

During one of her most lucid moments, Lisa asked me why God hadn't taken her yet and why He was letting her suffer this way. I told her that she had battled for so long, it was time for her to let God know she was ready to go. I told her it was time; she had suffered more than her fair share. But it wasn't enough to hear it from me, she needed to hear it from her dad, Peter. In Lisa's mind we all had to be ready. As difficult as it was, Peter said the words she had been waiting for. Whenever she woke up after this, she would ask why she was still here. It was heartbreaking to hear, and it was a question I also asked myself many times. By this stage, I was praying that God would let her slip away; we just wanted her free from pain.

On Friday 10th March 2017, the palliative doctor came to see Lisa. The caring night nurses had reported how much pain and discomfort she had been in through the night and how she had asked why she hadn't passed yet. He explained to Peter, Steven, Marianne

> We had to allow her full control right up to the finish line.

and me that, if Lisa was agreeable, it was time to intervene with palliative sedation. We were so relieved and grateful but agreed that the decision had to be Lisa's. Lisa had run her own race throughout this painful journey, and we had to allow her full control right up to the finish line, just as it should be.

In his usual way, the doctor pulled up a seat, got down to Lisa's level, touched her arm lightly and spoke her name. Lisa opened her eyes and said she had heard our conversation about sedation. The doctor told her that only she could make that decision. In true Lisa-style, she agreed but asked that he wait until she had eaten McDonalds. Being coeliac, Lisa hadn't had McDonalds for over eight years, but she had asked for it twice in her final week. When the doctor asked if there was anything else he could do for her, as quick as her old self Lisa said, "Yes, you could come with me," and we all had our final laugh with our beautiful, courageous girl.

We gave Lisa her final wish – McDonalds. Even though she could only manage two mouthfuls, it was enough to satisfy her craving and stick two fingers up to coeliac disease.

As hard as it is to admit, I felt so relieved that Lisa would be out of pain and that we wouldn't have to make any difficult decisions regarding her treatment. By 3pm she was sleeping soundly, lying down comfortably in bed for the first time in well over 12 months. The very sight of her at peace made us feel so at ease with where we were at. We didn't think about what was ahead; we were just in the moment and strangely enough content.

Although unsure of how long Lisa had left, we were advised that because she was young with a strong heart, she could last at least another week. We were not concerned. She was so peaceful and the palliative nurses so kind and caring. She was in the right place.

11 March 2017

On Saturday 11th March 2017, Peter and I woke up and I suggested that we tidy up Lisa's room. She was such an organised person and would have hated the room looking so cluttered. So we packed up most of her personal belongings in preparation for taking them home. When our family and close friends arrived, I immediately asked that we reduce the number of people gathered in the room as it could get noisy and hot. I just wanted the room to be as serene and as perfect as it could be. Steven and Marianne brought in Lisa's rock salt lamp and her music, which we played quietly throughout the day.

I had a feeling that Lisa wasn't going to be with us much longer.

The nurses, who we had grown to know and love, popped in as they finished their shift. They hugged Lisa and whispered their own wee private words to her, and then hugged us all before they went home, tears streaming. We thought they were sad that they were going to miss Lisa's passing. But we learned later that they were relieved to be going home as they didn't want to be there when she went. It would have been too hard to watch.

By 11pm the only people remaining were Peter, Marianne, me, our two best friends, Brian and Tom, and Lisa's two best friends, Bec and Sharon. Steven and my sister Bernie had taken Ava home to bed. Peter and I fully understood; we were all exhausted.

I decided to give Lisa a little freshen-up. I washed her face, hands and arms and applied some moisturiser. At 11.15pm I whispered to Lisa that there was a full moon. Because she was not great in the dark, I told her it would be the perfect night for her to go to heaven as she'd be guided by the light. At 11.45pm, Marianne and I were sitting holding Lisa's hands when Lisa took a small gasp of air. I asked Marianne if she thought this was the end. When Lisa had another small gasp of air, Marianne rushed to get Peter and the nurse. They reached the room in time to see Lisa take her last breath.

Our beautiful, brave girl passed away at 11:49pm on 11th March 2017.

She was no longer in pain, and her final day on earth could not have been more perfect.

We each took a private moment to say our goodbyes. I had to keep reminding myself that Lisa was at peace; it was the only way I could keep going. I will never forget the walk from Lisa's room to the hospital exit. I had the strongest feeling that I had left something behind ... Not my purse, my phone or my handbag ... It was our beautiful daughter.

Although I was surrounded by loved ones, that was the worst feeling on earth on the loneliest walk I've ever taken.

I knew there were others who had been walking with us so far, the Terminally Fabulous Rockstars, and after a day, I knew I had to let them know. I did it the only way I could – through the *Terminally Fabulous* Facebook page...

12/03/2017 Facebook post

Last night at 11.50pm, our gorgeous girl was wrapped in the wings of an angel and joined her friends and family in heaven. Lisa's passing was so peaceful, slipping away in her sleep without pain nor fear, just as we'd all prayed for. And more importantly, just as Lisa had wanted it. Her room had been calmly lit with her rock salt lamp, her music had been playing, and we'd held her hand and talked to her throughout the day. I just knew it was time.

I whispered to Lisa at 11pm that there was a full moon, which she loved. I told her it was there to light her way for her special journey. I washed her and freshened her up, and 50 minutes later she was gone. Our hearts are shattered into a thousand pieces. Lisa was one of the most generous souls to walk this earth. We were so blessed to have her in our lives.

One thing I know for sure is Lisa passed with so much love and support from around the world. You could feel the sincerity in every message and comment. Even though she was sleeping, we would tell her how her followers had really rallied behind her. I know in my heart of hearts this meant so, so much to her. Her supporters were her love and her passion. You gave her the strength to leave a legacy to be proud of.

Thank you, a million times over, for your never-ending support. Although the next few days will be one of our toughest challenges yet, I will be in touch in a couple of days to advise you how we're coping and where to from here.

Our sincerest love and thanks.

Geraldine Xox

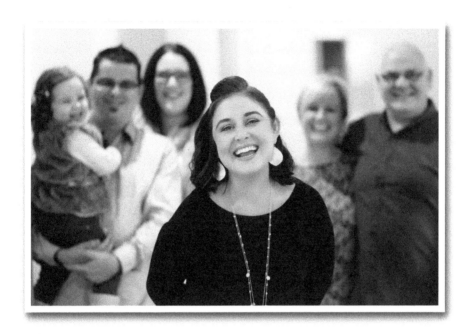

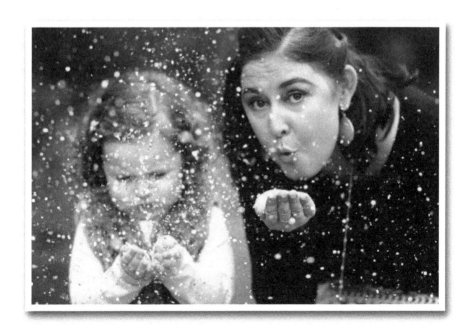

Walking With Grief

"Courage does not always roar.
Sometimes courage is that little
voice at the end of the day that
says I'll try again tomorrow."

~Mary Anne Radmacher

We were now moving from one nightmare into another: Grief...

Books, counsellors, friends and any piece ever written about grief will tell you about the stages of grief that you'll go through and in which order these stages occur. The truth is that these stages can happen at any time. They can be intertwined and happen when you least expect them.

For me, grief can be triggered by driving past a hospital, being in the gluten-free aisle of the local Woolworths, passing someone in the shopping mall with hospital greens on, and the worst, passing someone with a headscarf on and no eyebrows. This is when I feel like running over and grabbing this person and hugging the life right out of them. I want to make their pain go away. But how can I when I'm still in pain myself?

Since Lisa passed, we have fulfilled all her wishes and more, from the service in a quaint chapel by the water to a second service at home in Ireland with all our old friends and family. We talk to Ava daily about Lisa, generally because Ava has brought the subject of Lisa up and is looking for comfort. I know that Lisa will be looking down and wondering how she could have imagined our gorgeous baby girl would ever forget her. She loves her as much in death as she did in life.

As hard as it was for Peter, Steven and Marianne, they all returned to work after a couple of weeks of Lisa's passing and settled into their new normal. They each have their difficult days, but work keeps them focused and helps them move forward when needed. Our friends and family continue to be there for us, and Lisa's best friends have become part of our family. They never fail to sense when we need support and are always there with a call or a visit.

As for me, I'm still not sure how my new normal should look. Initially, I was weighed down by guilt. No matter how hard I tried, I could only remember the difficult times – the times Lisa and I had words. Well, Lisa had words and I had the lump in my throat. Every space of the house reminds me of Lisa, some good and some not so good. Lisa's bathroom still makes my heart skip a beat when I enter it. I don't think I will ever overcome this. Her room is sitting as she would have wanted it: clean, tidy and organised. Her urn is propped up on her bed, right where she belongs. It just feels right. I have even managed to organise her wardrobe, which was a massive achievement. I'm sure the day will come when I will be ready to give her beautiful clothes to someone who could use them. But I am nowhere close to being able to do that now. I continued with counselling until I felt strong enough to live my life without Lisa in it. By the time I accepted that Lisa was gone and never coming back, I could move forward one day at a time.

Twelve months on and I am now back at work. An old boss offered me a maternity cover position, and although I was extremely hesitant, I am so glad I accepted it. As strange as it sounds, I believe the reason I have enjoyed being at work so much is the fact that it's completely removed from the loss of Lisa. Nothing in the office is familiar – no hard-to-bear memories and pitiful looks. The longer I'm there, the more people get to learn about me and my family. Some have even approached me because they recognised me from the blog. They have all been so amazingly supportive but have also recognised the need for me to have some normality. I can laugh now, really laugh, and without the guilt I had felt for so long. I am now starting to recognise my old self again, something I didn't think would ever be possible.

Someone once told me that cancer would change us all for ever, and they were right. We have changed. Peter, Steven, Marianne, Ava and I have lived through something so tragic and heart-wrenching, how could life ever be the same for us? But we are here, living our new normal, which is exactly what Lisa would want for us. When we see a bright yellow butterfly, we say it's Lisa watching us. The brightest star in the sky will always be Lisa to us, and every time we have a glass of Mumm we are thinking of Lisa. The heart-stopping moments when we see an ambulance or hear the word 'cancer' become fewer and more bearable, but they will never disappear.

I have continued to update Lisa's blog and have kept her loyal followers informed with how we are coping. They continue to support me and the family just as they did Lisa. Their outpouring of love and concern never fails to amaze us, and we will always be grateful to them. They undoubtedly kept Lisa strong when she most needed it and have so generously helped us through our darkest days.

The encouragement they have given me whilst writing this book has been priceless. It is because of their support that I have taken up the opportunity to become a Guide for a beautiful charity called LifeCircle. As a Guide I will be able to support others caring for the terminally ill and will hopefully make their journey a little less daunting. A good listener and some advice from someone that has walked this journey was something that I would have found priceless, and I am determined to give back to those in need.

So where to from here? The reality is this was Lisa's story; it was Lisa's journey. For me to show Lisa the love and respect she deserves, I feel the time is right to end the blog. It will always be there. Lisa's crazy humour in her darkest days will never be lost. People will always be able to turn to it, but I feel the time is right to stop the updates.

I have new life goals now, and I can only move forward fully if I leave the past in the past. Does this mean I will stop thinking of Lisa every waking moment of every day? Absolutely not. But it does mean that I won't get lost in the grieving process to the point

Out of so much pain and suffering I'm hoping will come much good.

where I forget all my thoughts and ideas to help others and do all I can to make Lisa proud. Out of so much pain and suffering I'm hoping will come much good.

Our family has much to look forward to. We have a second grandchild on the way; Steven and Marianne will have their baby by the end of the year and we just can't wait. Did we all have that 'if only' moment when we heard their news? Of course we did. But the truth is, like Ava, our new baby will know everything about their beautiful Angel Aunt: her bravery, her love, her kindness and her humour. We will always talk of her with hearts full of pride. Rebecca, Lisa's best friend, is also having her first baby, a little boy, something that she so wished she was able to share with Lisa.

But the reality is that the day we lost Lisa our family circle grew. Out of despair came so much love. These beautiful babies will be so loved and protected by the most amazing guardian angel, and that will keep us going.

To those who continue to fight the good fight with cancer, stay strong and know you are not alone. Lisa would tell you to make the most of every good day, and if you are lucky enough to get the all-clear, speak to someone that can help you move on and enjoy life after your diagnosis. Grab your second chance and run with it.

And to those that are terminally fabulous, know that you are worth fighting for. On your darkest days talk to those you love. Lean on them and tell them how you feel. Most importantly, don't leave anything unsaid. You have this special opportunity to write your own ending. Grab it with both hands; you are what counts.

To those caring for your loved ones, please reach out and ask for help. Those around you don't know what to do. They know they want to help but don't know how. You may be the carer, but more importantly, you are still their loved one. Whatever the relationship make time to just be. Talk about everything that needs to be talked about. If your loved one wants to talk about death, talk about it. As hard as it is, it will only get harder at the end if you haven't discussed their dying wishes. Everyone deserves to have their final wishes met, and you will play a significant part in ensuring this happens.

Just as important, make sure you are looking after you. You cannot care for others if you do not care for yourself. Take time out when you can get it, go for a coffee, chat with a friend, go for a walk – anything that will help you clear your head. This is not an easy role. It will have you questioning everything you do and say. But just know that you are important too and you will get through this.

Love and gratitude always.

Geraldine

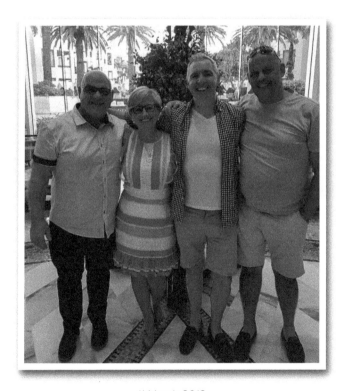

11 March 2018
Remembering Lisa on the first anniversary of her passing. Geraldine and Peter with Brian Carney and partner Tom Larsson at Palazzo Versace on the Gold Coast.

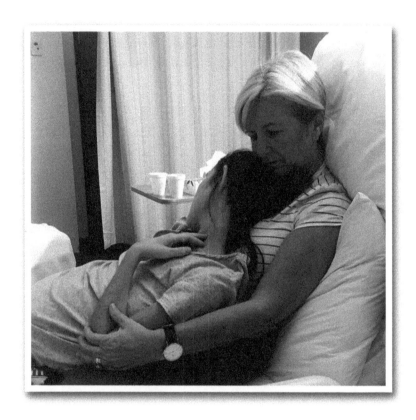

9 March 2017
In palliative care.

"I will treasure this photo until my dying day. When Lisa asked me
to get in behind her she was telling me we were as close as ever.
She'd been in so much pain, yet she slept like this for three hours.
I never moved an inch. I wanted time to stand still." – Geraldine

We knew that day you could not last
The time had come for you to pass.

You'd fought so hard to beat the pain
All we could do was watch in vain.

We held your hand as time slipped by
We didn't want for you to die.

Your heart was strong and you were tough
But we all knew you'd had enough.

The moon was full and shining bright
I whispered, "Lisa, it's the perfect night".

Those final gasps they let us know
The time had come for you to go.

We kissed your head and said goodbye
All we could do was sit and cry.

As we left your room and looked back at you
We thought our hearts had broken in two.

As years slipped by and times moved on
But we still struggle to accept you're gone.

So much news for you to hear
We try to remember you are always near.

Never forget how much we care
And living without you is hard to bear.

With heavy hearts we speak your name
But life without you is not the same.

Always loved and never forgotten, beautiful girl.

~Mummy and Daddy x

© Geraldine Magill

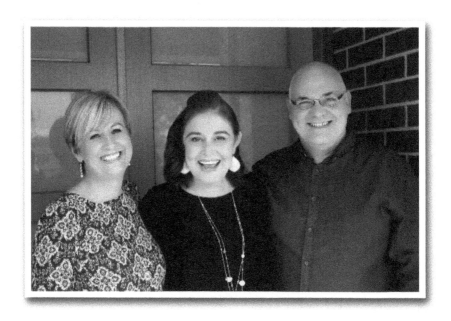

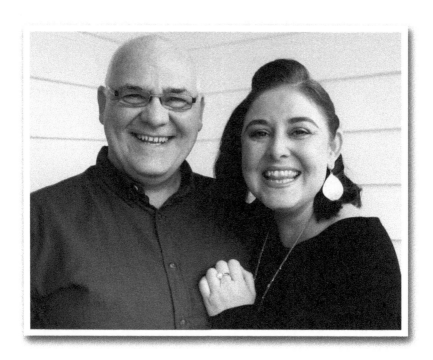

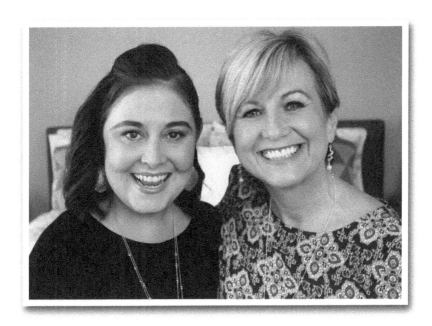

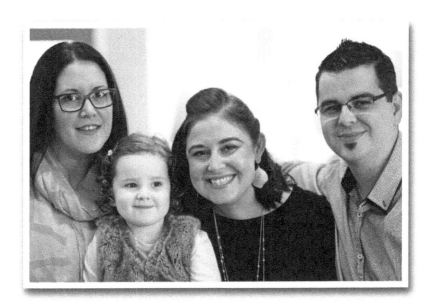

Cancer and Grief Support

> "Life isn't about waiting on the
> storm to pass; it's about learning
> to dance in the rain."
>
> ~Viviane Greene

Here are a few websites and links that can help children and adults who are dealing with cancer and bereavement in their lives.

AUSTRALIA

- www.cancer.org.au (To find a specialist look in the 'About cancer' tab)
- www.cancercouncil.com.au (Find useful support organisations, website and books for children and adults at www.cancercouncil.com. au/1374/uncategorized/when-a-parent-has-cancer-4)
- www.bereavementcare.com.au
- www.feelthemagic.org.au
- www.lifecircle.org.au
- www.australianclinicaltrials.gov.au
- www.grief.org.au
- www.kidshelp.com.au
- www.beyondblue.org.au
- www.lifeline.org.au

USA

- www.kidskonnected.org
- www.cancer.net (See the 'Coping With Cancer'/'Managing Emotions' tab for information on coping with grief and helping grieving children and teenagers)

UK

- www.riprap.org.uk
- www.winstonswish.org.uk
- www.childbereavementuk.org

CHARITIES

- www.dreams2live4.com.au
- www.rarecancers.org.au
- www.cancer.org.au

APP

Free patient support app
CAN.recall @ www.rarecancers.org.au

Contact the Author

You may read all of Lisa Magill's original blogs at the *Terminally Fabulous* website, where you can also contact her mother and co-author, Geraldine.

www.terminallyfabulous.com

Join the *Terminally Fabulous* community on Facebook:

www.facebook.com/terminallyfabulous

Lightning Source UK Ltd.
Milton Keynes UK
UKHW021156140321
380239UK00007B/149

9 780648 391715